PRAISE FOR *THE CA*

"We all aspire to exit our professions knowing that we mattered, that our work made a difference for generations to come. The stories and guidance in this book are just what we as nurse leaders need to help ensure that our legacies live on through those who follow us. Thank you, Kathy and Tim, for reminding us that the final gift from those who choose to lead is to provide a loving handoff to those who lead after us."

–Kathleen Sanford, DBA, RN, FACHE, FAAN
Senior Vice President & Chief Nursing Officer
Catholic Health Initiatives

"Malloch and Porter-O'Grady provide both a practical and inspirational guide that includes not only transition planning, but also the necessary skills nurse leaders must hone for the future. They define retirement not as a mere exit but as a thoughtful process that preserves our wisdom. The Career Handoff is a life manual for a career well-spent, setting the expectation that we must all give back to those who will continue to practice our profession."

–Pamela Austin Thompson, MS, RN, CENP, FAAN
Chief Executive Officer, American Organization of Nurse Executives
Senior Vice President, Chief Nursing Officer
American Hospital Association

"Reading this book was like having a conversation with the authors. Each chapter revealed a treasure of information that not only resulted in stretching my thinking about wisdom transfer across the generations, but also understanding what I need to do each day to become a better leader. Thank you, Kathy and Tim, for this extraordinary gift to our profession."

–Shirley Johnson, MS, MBA, RN
Senior Vice President and Chief Nursing and Patient Care Services Officer
City of Hope

THE CAREER HANDOFF

A Healthcare Leader's Guide to Knowledge & Wisdom Transfer Across Generations

KATHY MALLOCH, PHD, MBA, RN, FAAN

TIM PORTER-O'GRADY, DM, EDD,
SCD(H), APRN, FAAN, FACCWS

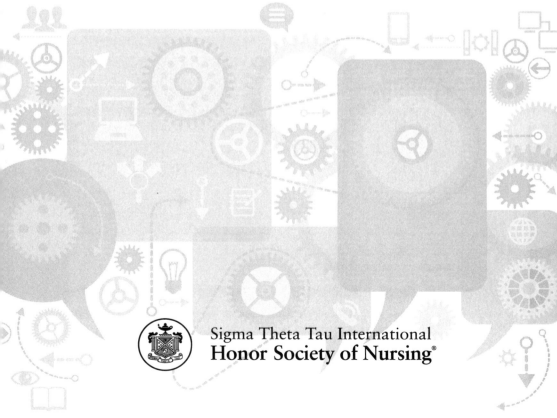

Sigma Theta Tau International
Honor Society of Nursing®

The Honor Society of Nursing, Sigma Theta Tau International (STTI) is a nonprofit organization founded in 1922 whose mission is to support the learning, knowledge, and professional development of nurses committed to making a difference in health worldwide. Members include practicing nurses, instructors, researchers, policymakers, entrepreneurs and others. STTI's 499 chapters are located at 698 institutions of higher education throughout Australia, Botswana, Brazil, Canada, Colombia, Ghana, Hong Kong, Japan, Kenya, Malawi, Mexico, the Netherlands, Pakistan, Portugal, Singapore, South Africa, South Korea, Swaziland, Sweden, Taiwan, Tanzania, United Kingdom, United States, and Wales. More information about STTI can be found online at www.nursingsociety.org.

Sigma Theta Tau International
550 West North Street
Indianapolis, IN, USA 46202

To order additional books, buy in bulk, or order for corporate use, contact Nursing Knowledge International at 888.NKI.4YOU (888.654.4968/US and Canada) or +1.317.634.8171 (outside US and Canada).

To request a review copy for course adoption, e-mail solutions@nursingknowledge.org or call 888.NKI.4YOU (888.654.4968/US and Canada) or +1.317.634.8171 (outside US and Canada).

To request author information, or for speaker or other media requests, contact Marketing, Honor Society of Nursing, Sigma Theta Tau International at 888.634.7575 (US and Canada) or +1.317.634.8171 (outside US and Canada).

ISBN: 9781940446509
EPUB ISBN: 9781940446516
PDF ISBN: 9781940446523
MOBI ISBN: 9781940446530

Library of Congress Cataloging-in-Publication data

The career handoff : a healthcare leader's guide to knowledge & wisdom transfer across generations / [edited by] Kathy Malloch, Timothy Porter-O'Grady.
    p. ; cm.
Includes bibliographical references and index.
    ISBN 978-1-940446-50-9 (print : alk. paper) -- ISBN 978-1-940446-51-6 (epub) -- ISBN 978-1-940446-52-3 (pdf) -- ISBN 978-1-940446-53-0 (mobi)
    I. Malloch, Kathy, editor. II. Porter-O'Grady, Timothy, editor. III. Sigma Theta Tau International, issuing body.
    [DNLM: 1. Nursing Staff--education. 2. Intergenerational Relations. 3. Mentors. 4. Retirement. 5. Staff Development. WY 18]
    RT86.5
    362.17'3--dc23
                        2015036232

First Printing, 2015

Publisher: Dustin Sullivan

Acquisitions Editor: Emily Hatch

Editorial Coordinator: Paula Jeffers

Cover Designer: Rebecca Batchelor

Interior Design/Page Layout: Rebecca Batchelor

Principal Book Editor: Carla Hall

Development and Project Editor: Jennifer Lynn

Copy Editor: Charlotte Kughen

Proofreader: Todd Lothery

Indexer: Jane Palmer

DEDICATION

This book is dedicated to our colleagues who willingly and graciously share their wisdom every day to make the world a better place. You brighten our days and make it easier for others to learn more quickly, repeat fewer errors, and allow more time for this special handoff work to nourish not only our young but all generations.

ACKNOWLEDGMENTS

No feat is ever accomplished in isolation, and this book is no exception. My availability to write and consult within healthcare continues to be supported by many people and two in particular: Bryan, my husband of nearly 30 years, and Tim, the best colleague and friend one could ever hope to have. Bryan provides unconditional support for the work I am doing, and for that I will be eternally grateful. Tim continues to be the best there is in every venue we work in. He is incredibly smart, patient, and focused. Finally, our chapter authors have been a delight to work with; some are very experienced writers and some are first-time writers. Each chapter author embraced this work with passion for the message and dedication to creating an excellent product.

–Kathy

What a great opportunity this has been to share with great colleagues and work together on a project that focuses on continuing to build the future of our profession. I have been fortunate to be associated with the best nurses in every arena of practice, and I'm grateful for the experience. I am especially thankful to my co-author, Kathy Malloch, for her wisdom, patience, and kindness on the professional and personal journey we have taken together during the past 20 years—it has been a great collaboration. To Mark Ponder, my partner in life for the past 38 years, I can only say how much my life has been blessed because you have traveled with me. And to my colleagues, young and old, emerging and retiring, I am eternally grateful for your continuing inspiration and contribution to my learning and for enriching my appreciation for the profession we love so deeply.

–Tim

ABOUT THE AUTHORS

KATHY MALLOCH, PHD, MBA, RN, FAAN

Kathy Malloch is president of KMLS, LLC, professor of practice at ASU College of Nursing and Health Innovation, clinical professor at The Ohio State University College of Nursing, and clinical consultant at API Healthcare, A GE Healthcare company. A recognized expert in leadership and the development of evidence-based systems for patient care, her uncanny focus on accountability and results is the hallmark of her practice. Her expertise has been useful to many organizations across the country. A nationally known writer and speaker, Malloch has been a registered nurse for more than 40 years. Malloch has published extensively in proctored health journals. She is a frequent presenter and author on leadership topics. Malloch served as the first program director for the Arizona State University, College of Nursing and Health Innovation, Master's in Healthcare Innovation program. Most recently, she and Tim Porter-O'Grady created the Executive DNP Program at OSU-College of Nursing, Columbus, Ohio. Malloch is the designer of the Expert Nurse Estimation Patient Classification System (ENEPCS), an innovative model to integrate the role of the professional nurse in daily nurse-patient staffing to achieve the best outcomes.

TIM PORTER-O'GRADY, DM, EDD, SCD(H), APRN, FAAN, FACCWS

Tim Porter-O'Grady is senior partner with Tim Porter-O'Grady Associates, Inc., professor of practice at ASU College of Nursing and Health Innovation, clinical professor and leadership scholar at The Ohio State University College of Nursing, and adjunct professor at Emory University School of Nursing. Porter-O'Grady has been involved in healthcare for 44 years and has held roles from clinical provider to senior executive in a variety of American healthcare settings. Porter-O'Grady is currently senior partner of an international healthcare consulting firm in Atlanta, Georgia, USA (Tim Porter-O'Grady Associates Inc.). Since 1991 he has been specializing in health futures, organizational innovation, conflict and change, and complex health service delivery models. He has consulted nationally on health reform during both the Clinton and Obama administrations. He is noted for his work on shared governance models, clinical leadership, conflict, innovation, complex systems, and health futures. Porter-O'Grady holds academic scholar positions at two major universities (Arizona State University and The Ohio State University), and he is a registered mediator and arbitrator and an APRN wound specialist. He is a clinical volunteer wound specialist practicing at Mercy Care Clinics for the Homeless in Atlanta. He has published 23 books (8 have won *AJN* Book of the Year awards) and more than 200 proctored journal articles. Porter-O'Grady has been called an enthusiastic, energetic, and inspiring presenter and teacher and has made more than 500 appearances as a lecturer at both U.S. and international venues.

CONTRIBUTING AUTHORS

GREGORY CROW, EDD, RN

Gregory Crow is emeritus professor and former director of graduate programs in leadership, case management, and education at California State University, Sonoma. Crow has more than 35 years of professional nursing practice in a variety of roles and settings. His administrative and leadership positions have included clinical supervisor, director of nursing, and assistant hospital administrator for patient care services for a multihospital system. Crow's current positions are senior consultant with Tim Porter-O'Grady Associates for 20 years, and adjunct professor and director of the Vietnam Nurse Project (www.usfca.edu/nursing/Vietnam) at the University of San Francisco. Crow consults internationally in organizational and systems development, creating motivating work environments, transformational change, and the implementation of shared governance systems. He presents on these topics at state, national, and international conferences. Crow's publications appear in a wide variety of professional nursing journals and textbooks.

JANICE GANANN, MED, PCC

Janice Ganann is managing director at JLP and Associates, LLC. Ganann possesses more than 20 years of experience in leadership roles, and her expertise includes leadership effectiveness, organizational development, succession planning, and organizational communications. Prior to founding her own consulting practice, Ganann led the executive talent function for Banner Health. In that position, her primary responsibilities included building the leadership pipeline. She skillfully managed Banner Health's succession planning process. In addition, she led the physician leadership development strategies within the entire system. Ganann's broad-based experience includes executive coaching for senior leaders and teams that are committed to reaching the highest levels of business results and personal satisfaction. She supports people in reaching new levels of achievement by challenging them with an unwavering commitment to personal development. Ganann holds a master's degree in educational leadership from Northern Arizona University in Flagstaff, Arizona, and a bachelor's degree in communications from the University of Iowa in Iowa City, Iowa.

JANELLE KRUEGER, MBA, BSN, RN, CCRN

Janelle Krueger is senior director of Clinical Operations at the Hospital Division of Kindred Healthcare. In her 20 years with Kindred, Krueger has served in corporate- and regional-level positions in clinical, quality, administrative, and informatics departments. She has extensive experience in critical care and operational system management. She excels at program management for patient classification systems and has a passion for empowering and valuing nurses through workload management initiatives and the promotion of safe patient care. She has co-authored a chapter on patient classification systems in a nursing textbook. Krueger has comprehensive knowledge and experience in regulatory compliance, patient safety initiatives, clinical information systems, and hospital administrative roles. She received her nursing degree at Viterbo University in LaCrosse, Wisconsin, and her MBA at the University of Phoenix.

MARY LOCKHART, PHD, MS

Mary Lockhart is system program manager for quality at PeaceHealth. She is an experienced healthcare manager with expertise in leading patient experience and health education programs. She has an extensive background in operational and strategic planning and patient-centered innovations in care delivery, and her experience spans nonprofit health-care systems, university settings, and community organizations. She has achieved notable results in all these environments. Lockhart's strengths include creating effective partnerships with diverse stakeholders and transforming vision into effective action. For the past 8 years, Lockhart has been a system program manager for Quality at PeaceHealth, a non-profit healthcare system. Prior to joining PeaceHealth, Lockhart was co-director of Health Education Services for Kaiser Permanente in the Northwest Region, where she managed operational functions focused on the delivery of health education information, training, and consulta-tion to patients and other clients. Lockhart holds a PhD in community health and a master's degree in counseling psychology.

ADRIENNE LYONS, MSN, RN

Adrienne Lyons is a clinical consultant at Kindred Healthcare. She is a registered nurse with more than 30 years' experience in caring for criti-cally ill adults. She currently serves as a clinical consultant with Kindred Healthcare's Hospital Division. From 1999 until 2012 she was the se-nior director of Clinical Operations for the Kindred Central Region and was responsible for implementation and maintenance of clinical pro-grams and regulatory compliance in transitional care hospitals. In 2012 she assumed a consultant status in order to pursue a lifelong dream of earning a doctorate. She enrolled in the Doctor of Nursing Practice pro-gram at Loyola University Chicago with a focus on patient safety and outcomes management. She was awarded the DNP degree in November 2014. Her specialty is cognition and delirium management in the criti-cally ill adult. Lyons is a member of the American Association of Crit-ical-Care Nurses, is active in Chicago area initiatives to end childhood hunger, and participates in food distribution for the local food pantry.

JENNIFER MENSIK, PHD, MBA, RN, NEA-BC, FAAN

Jennifer Mensik is an instructor at Arizona State University and director of Professional Practice at Banner Health Ironwood Medical Center. She earned a PhD in nursing from the University of Arizona College of Nursing with a major in health systems and a minor in public administration from the Eller Business College. Mensik has authored and coauthored numerous publications, including the books *The Nurse's Step-by-Step Guide to Transitioning to the Professional Nurse Role* (2015), *Lead, Drive & Thrive in the System* (2014), *and The Nurse Manger's Guide to Innovative Staffing* (2013). Mensik led the development of the Professional Nursing Practice Framework, which is now used in all Banner Health hospitals and has been adopted by other non-Banner Health hospitals and medical centers nationally. Mensik was named Alumni of the Year for the University of Arizona College of Nursing in 2010. Mensik has served as the president of the Arizona Nurses Association and as second vice president on the Board of Directors for the American Nurses Association. Additionally, she held the role of governor of nursing practice for the Western Institute of Nursing.

APRIL MYERS, MBA, FACHE

April Myers is market chief executive officer at Kindred Healthcare. Myers has more than 20 years of hospital executive leadership experience with hospitals across the United States. She currently serves as the market chief executive officer for three free-standing Southern California hospitals that are part of Kindred Healthcare, a Fortune 500 healthcare services company and a top-85 private employer in the United States. Her passion is centered on the triple-bottom-line philosophy of employee satisfaction, patient satisfaction, and financial profitability while maximizing employee engagement, operational efficiency, organizational excellence, and team building. Myers earned her MBA from Louisiana State University and earned her bachelor's of business administration from Midwestern State University. She is also certified as a fellow of the American College of Healthcare Executives.

OLIVIA QUIST, MA

Olivia Quist is associate broker at Russ Lyons Real Estate. She is an example of a lifelong learner. Growing up on a ranch in New Mexico, she spent many hours with her father, learning from experience about farming and ranching. At the University of New Mexico, she majored in speech and drama as an undergraduate and obtained her master's of art in English literature. She taught for several years in Albuquerque and then moved to Phoenix where she became a real estate agent and has had a successful career for 35 years. She believes every situation provides an opportunity to learn, both in formal classes and from life experiences. Quist is now in her 80s, and she continues to take university-level classes online.

JENNIFER SCHOMBURG, MHA, MA

Jennifer Schomburg is chief operating officer at Northwest Medical Center in Tucson, Arizona. For the past 14 years, Schomburg has served in administrative positions in both the acute and post-acute sectors with HCA, UHS, Fremont Emergency Services, Kindred Healthcare, and CHS. She is experienced in leading large expansion projects, including opening new hospitals and leading teams charged with acquisitions, mergers, process improvement, service line development, and strategic planning. Schomburg is passionate about bringing staff of diverse backgrounds and strengths together and moving them to excellence. She believes in the power of leadership by being inclusive and in developing leaders at all levels of an organization. She received her master's of healthcare administration and master's of philosophy from the University of Missouri-Columbia.

DOROTHY SISNEROS, MS, MBA, FAACVPR

Dorothy Sisneros is managing partner at Thunderbird Leadership Consulting, LLC, and partner of Language of Caring, LLC. Sisneros has been involved in healthcare and education for more than 30 years and brings her experience as leader, executive coach, organization development consultant, and speaker to clients across the United States. She currently leads the Language of Caring's Client Services and Implementation Team and is also a managing partner in Thunderbird Leadership Consulting. Sisneros has worked with organizations on systemwide initiatives as an internal leader and as a partner and consultant. She knows the power of effective teams in the workplace, and she is skilled at guiding leaders to engage the wisdom of employees and to build on their strengths to help them move to the next level of performance. She moves people and ideas to excellence, focusing teams to meet their goals and transforming complex ideas and processes into positive outcomes. Sisneros received her MS from the University of Wisconsin-LaCrosse, MBA from the University of Phoenix, and BS from the University of Arizona.

AMY STEINBINDER, PHD, RN, NE-BC

Amy Steinbinder is managing partner at Thunderbird Leadership Consulting. Steinbinder's 11-year consulting practice builds on her 30 years of proven leadership experience in healthcare organizations. She is an established organizational effectiveness consultant and executive coach who is well versed in leading large-scale change, cycles of innovation, and cultural transformation using complex adaptive systems, appreciative inquiry, and positive deviance principles. She is co-founder and principal of Thunderbird Leadership Consulting. Clients have included Arizona Hospital and Healthcare Association, Adelante Healthcare, Presbyterian Emergency Physicians, Health Services Advisory Group, Kindred Healthcare, Scripps, Maricopa Corporate College, ProHealth Care, and ProHealth Solutions. Steinbinder worked in the Banner Health System for more than 20 years in various roles, including service excellence administrator, patient safety officer, senior director of nursing systems, director of professional practice, and organizational development consultant. She had responsibility for patient experience, leadership development, quality improvement, root-cause analysis, instructional design, and Magnet redesignation.

TABLE OF CONTENTS

FOREWORD

This book opens up ways for an enlightened transmission of knowledge and wisdom from one generation to another. Those who are ignorant of the past are condemned to repeat failures and ignore past enlightened practices and successes. By making transitions from one generation of nurses to another more explicit and thoughtful, these authors contribute to a more enlightened and progressive future. The ironic, wise statement "It is not change that is difficult … it is the transition" is a central message of this inspiring book. Once you can survey a change that has already occurred, the difficulty is usually behind you. How we cope with, plan for, and civilize transitions from positions can ensure a better future. This is especially true for transitions from professional leadership positions into retirement, where the retiring person holds years of institutional wisdom and tradition that are crucial for effective transitions within a complex practice such as healthcare. It is here that attention to transitions and transmission of lessons learned over time become so crucial for sustaining excellence and a better future.

Even though we are in the midst of major and multiple stages of transition into what is diversely understood as an age of postmodernism(s), we are also still very much in the grips of the Enlightenment tradition. In the Enlightenment tradition, science is valued, and the past is viewed as something to be overturned or at least changed. Ironically, the Enlightenment tradition is known as the "anti-tradition tradition" (Shils, 1981). Shils points out that the Enlightenment tradition misunderstands the very notion of tradition. Anti-traditionalism is itself a tradition. For example, the Enlightenment tradition highly values progress made through rationality and empirical science. There is also a value for expressive individualism, where individuals must discover their own originality and talents and not be a passive recipient of society's influences and dictates on their individuality. This makes it difficult within the Enlightenment tradition to plan for and develop practices of transmission of wisdom, insights, and experiential learning gained in any living tradition. Without planned transitions, institutional progress and regressions are overlooked.

The Stanford Encyclopedia of Philosophy (Bristow, 2011) describes the later Enlightenment tradition, citing Kant as a leading figure:

> Kant defines "enlightenment" as humankind's release from its self-incurred immaturity; "immaturity is the inability to use one's own understanding without the guidance of another." Enlightenment is the process of undertaking to think for oneself, to employ and rely on one's own intellectual capacities in determining what to believe and how to act. Enlightenment philosophers from across the geographical and temporal spectrum tend to have a great deal of confidence in humanity's intellectual powers, both to achieve systematic knowledge of nature and to serve as an authoritative guide in practical life. This confidence is generally paired with suspicion or hostility toward other forms or carriers of authority (such as tradition, superstition, prejudice, myth and miracles), insofar as these are seen to compete with the authority of reason. (para. 3)

Even to the postmodern ear, this self-reliance, suspicion of "truths from the past" experience is easily devalued. Most professionals recognize the extremity of Enlightenment's individualistic view that one does not need past wisdom, or even history, to avoid the mistakes of the past or to sustain progress that has been hard-won. Self-reliance is necessary but not sufficient for growth and progress at the individual or institutional level. This book thoughtfully engages the topic of passing on insights, wisdom, and institutional history and culture.

Those who are formally retiring from an organization have much to offer, especially if their offerings are tempered with a recognition of excellent practices and an accurate memory of past failures and wrong turns that have since been corrected. No organization can progress if all past learning—successful and failed experiments—is forgotten. The authors of this book thoughtfully examine the responsibilities of both giving and receiving front-line wisdom and mistakes of the past. Learning organizations will do well to thoughtfully consider the major transition occurring as baby boomers retire and carry with them the memory of significant improvement in quality and safety, as well as expensive mistakes. In the past, for example, nurses experienced almost unlimited responsibility but had limited authority within healthcare organizations. Nurses were among the few predominantly female professions that were not clamoring for more responsibility during the equal rights phase of feminism. Nurses need to include the lessons and victories gained by equal rights feminists. And equally important is the later wave of feminism that recognized the knowledge and wisdom embedded in caring practices, such as nursing, social work, teaching, and more. To continue with an oppositional version of feminism that mimicked the male strategies of leadership and "powers over" would continue to reinforce strategies of patriarchy and authoritarianism, while all but ignoring authoritative and empowering leadership and power-use needed by all disciplines organized to care for and nurture others.

The reader has much to look forward to in reading the reflections on lessons learned and institutional knowledge passed on, as well as impediments to progressive improved care for patient populations and society in general. The art of listening and receiving the wisdom embedded in practice is aptly discussed by Jennifer Mensik and Jennifer Schomburg. Effective transitions require more than reflections on the past, as this book carefully points out: A focus on the future and needed new visions must also be considered. Learning from past successes and failure is essential to transforming the future of healthcare. This book makes many insightful contributions toward improving nursing and healthcare delivery. It deserves to be read by all nurses, particularly those in positions of leadership.

–Patricia Benner, PhD, RN, FAAN
Professor Emerita in the Department of Social and
Behavioral Sciences at the University of California, San Francisco
Former Senior Scholar at the Carnegie Foundation
for the Advancement of Teaching

REFERENCES

Bristow, W. (2011, Summer). Enlightenment. In E. N. Zalta (Ed.), *The Stanford encyclopedia of philosophy*. Retrieved from http://plato.stanford.edu/archives/sum2011/entries/enlightenment/

Shils, E. (1981). *Tradition*. Chicago, IL: University of Chicago Press.

INTRODUCTION

"Let us each and all realizing the importance of our influence on others—stand shoulder to—and not alone in good cause."
—Florence Nightingale

As seasoned writers, Tim and I believe it is important to share not only our leadership journeys, but also our writing journeys as one of the ways we can pay it forward for the nursing profession. Both of us have incredible mentors, both currently and throughout our careers, who have made our journeys richer and more enjoyable. We believe all professionals working to be better and to make the nursing profession better should have similar support and experiences. During our careers, we have willingly shared our knowledge and content with individuals along the way, and now we want to share in a larger way so that succession planning in nursing and healthcare enjoys a more scientific and personal foundation.

This book is intended first to share wisdom that we believe will help others in their journeys and second to engage authors—some new to the writing experience and some seasoned—to collaborate with us in this work. Our hope is that every nurse will find at least one nugget in these chapters that will be helpful or, even better, inspirational to their professional careers. We also hope this book inspires our colleagues to discover additional ways to advance the nursing profession and share that new information.

We are honored to have Patricia Benner write a Foreword for us. Benner has been a long-time friend and colleague who has inspired us to reflect on our journey from novice clinicians to experts in nursing and to always be the best we can be. We need to reflect on personal knowledge, recognize our value, and not be afraid to share our often too silent wisdom with our colleagues. We can all look to Benner as the pinnacle role model for excellence in nursing practice.

The chapters in this book take you on a journey that begins with the seedlings that inspired this book to the final chapter that reminds us of our responsibility to protect and support the future of the nursing profession and the nurses who will lead that charge. At the end of each chapter you will find a featured titled "Personal Application." We encourage you to review the key points and questions to assist you in your journey to both give and receive the wisdom of others.

> Chapter 1, "Intentional Sharing of Knowledge & Wisdom," introduces the topic of wisdom sharing, coaching, and mentoring as an ethical responsibility of nurses. The development of dialogue into a printed reality is chronicled along with experiences from the authors. The message is that purposeful and formal succession planning and handing off of wisdom and experiences are critical to the historical evolution of the nursing profession.

> Chapter 2, "Preparation for Knowledge & Wisdom Transfer," presents information on how to determine what really matters. As accomplished professionals, we often believe that everything we do and have said should be carefully enshrined and saved for the ages. On the other, more realistic, hand, we also think about situations—such as cleaning out our mother's house after her passing—and know that not everything is or should be kept for the future. The authors provide guidelines for this filtering process that guide readers to seek out the valuable wisdom that will continue to impact the future in a positive way and to gently put aside that which is no longer relevant.

Chapter 3, "Essential Business Knowledge," is about the perennial journey to discover and document the value of nursing practice. In this chapter, the tangible tools and competencies to fully engage in your work are presented. This chapter also includes information on spreadsheets, data management, and balanced scorecards.

Chapter 4, "Essential Business Relationships," continues the sharing of business value creation for the nursing profession. The focus is on the intangible competencies of relationship building, ways to gain organizational knowledge, the importance of lifelong reading, and collaboration and trust building with financial staff. An interview with Tim Porter-O'Grady on nursing value concludes this chapter.

In Chapter 5, "The Art and Science of Knowledge & Wisdom Transfer," the authors, who are members of Generation X, provide guidance on the art and science of receiving knowledge from other generations and capitalizing on every generation's perspectives. The authors emphasize the importance of storytelling, different styles of learning, generational characteristics, the impact of technology and the Internet, and the overall challenges in managing large amounts of data and information. The chapter includes a list of helpful tips for receiving information, knowledge, wisdom, and insight. Finally, the chapter concludes with a discussion of the importance of finding common ground across generations.

Chapter 6, "Strategies for Successful Knowledge & Wisdom Transfer," focuses on learning how to assure that our mentoring processes include personal styles and outcomes of relationships. The six strategies to enhance relationships provide useful tools to make the best of mentoring relationships. The authors explain the importance of mentors not merely passing on information but also passing on information with interpretations that will accommodate the new generations. Interviews with Marlene Kramer, Rhonda Anderson, and Ann Van Slyck enrich and demonstrate the value of the six strategies.

In Chapter 7, "Lifelong Learning and Giving," the authors approach wisdom sharing from the perspective of lifelong learning beyond traditional schooling and on into retirement. The challenges of pursuing doctoral education when one is in his/ her 60s are shared from a reflective and experiential perspective. One of the authors, Olivia Quist, is an amazing member of the Mature generation. She shares experiences of learning and wisdom sharing that continually enhance her own knowledge as well as the knowledge of others. Multiple sources of online adult education are presented to assist readers in developing their personal goals for incredibly rich learning in the most convenient way possible.

Chapter 8, "Leaving Nursing Better Than You Found It," is the final chapter and provides a rich reflection for all of us—nurses and those representing other professions—to stop and reflect on what have we done for our professions. Ultimately, we want nursing to be in a better place than when we entered the profession. The authors offer both challenges and meaningful strategies to make this a reality.

Roxanne Spitzer contributed an Afterword to this book. Although we have never included an Afterword in our other publications, we felt it would be appropriate to have a nursing legend share thoughts on the importance of wisdom management and sharing. We value her incredible experiences in nursing and healthcare and treasure her friendship throughout the years.

The intent of this book is about engagement with the profession and with our colleagues in a way that nursing is enhanced and that all nurses are aware of contributions of all generations. We hope you find the Personal Application feature helpful and that it will serve as a reference you access numerous times in the future.

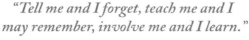

*"Tell me and I forget, teach me and I
may remember, involve me and I learn."*
—Benjamin Franklin

1
INTENTIONAL SHARING OF KNOWLEDGE & WISDOM

KATHY MALLOCH, PHD, MBA, RN, FAAN
TIM PORTER-O'GRADY, DM, EDD, SCD(H), APRN, FAAN, FACCWS

CHAPTER OBJECTIVES

Describe the compelling drivers to formalize handing off of
intellectual property.

Define the basic elements of mentorship and succession.

Clarify the elements, characteristics, and dynamics of the
mentoring relationship as a part of the process of leadership succession.

Develop insights for determining the personal commitment
and role in transitioning, mentoring, and succession.

Every year, Tim and I schedule time for a retreat to plan what we are going to focus on in the next year. We select a special place where we can both think and play and do something special. At our latest retreat at the Ojai Valley Inn & Spa in California, we found ourselves wondering how many more revisions of our work we could do—and how much longer our ideas and strategies would be relevant for healthcare organizations. And then came the even tougher question: What would happen to our textbooks? Would *Quantum Leadership* just sail into the sunset? We humbly wanted the information that would be meaningful to future generations not to be lost; we did not want future generations to rediscover what we had already identified and shared. These questions got us to think about how to hand off our successful ideas to younger colleagues and selectively discard that which is no longer relevant. From that conversation, we began to strategize and learn about how to hand off knowledge and wisdom to younger generations, and this book is a result of those ideas.

We realized from our consulting practices that highly successful professionals are often reluctant to consider retirement, and many people avoid the thought of moving away from active engagement with colleagues in sharing knowledge and wisdom. It is even more challenging to figure out how to hand off or give one's intellectual property to another colleague. As an unprecedented number of baby boomers move closer to retirement, there is much to share with succeeding generations. There is also some content or intellectual property that might not be applicable in future generations. We believe a formalized process for sharing and designating intellectual property and products would be helpful to not only our baby boomer colleagues but also to other generations of colleagues.

THE NEED FOR GENERATIONAL SHARING

Our professional consulting focus has been on the importance of leadership and in helping others to learn as much as possible about leadership—to embrace new ideas to become the most successful leaders possible. Our belief has always been that everyone is a leader, regardless of whether they have a formal leadership title. Whenever two individuals are together, one person begins the dialogue or movement in the simplest way, and leadership is evident. Each one of us has some special knowledge and expertise that future generations should or might want. Creating a culture as well as validating the science that assists others in handing off and nourishing our colleagues with our wisdom is important to both of us. Cultivating a culture of giving to others with minimal expectations of receiving something in return will allow future generations to grow and move on with what is vital to them. Our focus has shifted from figuring out what to give and how to instruct them to "love our stuff" to identifying interested colleagues and turning our work over to them to sort out and retain what is deemed valuable. It is also time for us to get out of the way of future leaders and shift from driving the boat to creating a safe space for others learning how to manage the boat's journey!

Soon after our retreat, I was invited to keynote a leadership summit group; my focus was on this topic of generational sharing. Participants at this meeting included successful professionals from three generations, including chief executive officers, nurse executives, consultants, real estate executives, and physicians. As part of the keynote, I presented the plan Tim and I developed to hand off two of our books (see the feature that follows) and the discussion began to flow. Participants were highly interested in learning more and becoming involved in advancing the science of both giving and receiving intellectual property and the wisdom of ages.

HANDING OFF OUR PUBLICATIONS

After many years of writing books and revising those books, Tim and I wondered what would happen to our book content when we were really finished writing. So, after some thought, we decided to be proactive and formally pass on the writings.

Over the course of our careers we had had many excellent students and colleagues; we selected two who we thought embraced our philosophy about innovation and leadership *and* had a track record for getting things done. We asked Dr. Dan Weberg and Dr. Sandra Davidson if they would be interested in taking on the work of combining our evidence-based practice (EBP) books with our *Innovation Leadership* book to make one "Innovation–Evidence Dynamic" book. They were extremely excited and ready to set up and pursue a plan to make this happen. Our next step was to contact the publisher and present our idea.

The publisher developed a contract, and Tim and I reviewed and approved it. Then it went to Dan and Sandra as the new lead authors. For this new book, Dan and Sandra would be the lead authors while Tim and I followed them. In the next edition, only Dan and Sandra will be listed as authors, and Tim and I will be contributors as the new authors deem necessary. Dan and Sandra skillfully took the chapter content from both books, rearranged it, added new chapters, and deleted those they thought were less relevant in today's healthcare world.

Interestingly, this process seemed complicated when we began; however, with the highly professional new authors, the book has taken on a life of its own and is due to be published in the fall of 2015. We are excited to see the new book and know that Dan and Sandra will have exceeded our expectations.

Reflecting on these ideas, we created a book proposal with the interested retreat participants. We now had a team of wisdom experts to join us on this journey and, most importantly, the authors represented three generations of interested professionals. We realized quickly that the importance of sharing generational wisdom was significant and that there was much interest from younger generations in learning more about our work and how to keep the useful knowledge alive and contemporary. Rather than seeing ourselves as the *fading generation*, it is time to see ourselves as a generation who now has much to share with the younger generations! We believe we created a talented team of wisdom managers to assist in this work.

Further dialogue with the contributing authors provided clarification and enhancement of our ideas and solidified the importance of documenting and sharing generational wisdom, successes, and strategies that we would not repeat. We believe formalizing this process and providing guidelines for colleagues will be an important contribution to professional nursing practice. Each one of our authors has included specific discussion on what the handoff is, some practical tips for sharing knowledge, and exemplars to demonstrate personal experiences (and, of course, some irreverent humor; we all need to laugh and enjoy the nuances of our journey!).

This book reflects our commitment to professional coaching, mentoring, and assuring that our young nurses are not chewed up by the system but are supported proactively. Mentoring is a vital professional behavior and an ethical obligation to our profession; we need to nourish our young rather than engage in the proverbial "eating our young." In the next section, we share our personal and scholarly connections to the art and science of mentoring.

LIFE JOURNEY: MEMBERSHIP IN THE PROFESSION

Transitions and transformations are a fundamental part of the journey of life. Naturally, as we age and grow, we gather information, skill, insight, and wisdom that accumulate and aggregate in a way that becomes a part of our characters and personalities. As professionals, one of the most important considerations is the responsibility that membership in the nursing profession brings. Who we are and what we are become a part of our professional identity such that our person and profession become one and the same thing (Malloch & Porter-O'Grady, 2010). As we journey through our careers and our lives and are recognized as professional nurses, we essentially become the "person of the nurse." As professionals, we integrate our work, our relationships, and our individual persona in a way that creates the frame for who we are and provides the substance of the image we present to the world. Consider a notice you might see in a newspaper about the appointment of a position to an administrative or public role—the writer acknowledges the relationship between the person and profession by identifying the particular individual as a "physician." However, when a nurse is appointed in a similar fashion to an administrative or public role, he or she will more frequently be identified as a "former nurse." For the physician the identity is singular; for the nurse the same identity is dual (a nurse is a job different from the administrative or public role and, therefore, cannot be identified in singular terms).

SAGE INSIGHT SHARED ACROSS THE GENERATIONS

We have had many opportunities to work with a number of organizations in helping to increase awareness of the many "sage" resources within those organizations. Often, the usual obligations of work overtake the value of reflection on past experiences, special skills, organizational tenure, insights, and wisdom gained from many years of providing healthcare services. In their haste to embrace contemporary challenges and opportunities for innovation, leaders often forget to access the tremendous acumens and talents of the more mature and long-tenured contributors in their midst. At the same time, those with gifts and wisdom to share need also to be available to their colleagues and new members of the professional staff in ways that are open, responsive, and engaging.

A positive and renewing attitude that generates a sense of accomplishment and confidence provides a firm foundation out of which connections between a mentor and mentee can stimulate more positive relationships, meaningful interactions, and learning that can occur only between generations. Handing off knowledge to successive generations implies commitment and communication with those among us who have fresh ideas and different perspectives that need to be in-cluded in the dialogue among generations. As consultants with long tenure, we have been able to bring insights from outside the organization that may have already been available inside the organization, but leaders were often tied up with the challenges of the day in ways that didn't make the same important insights easily visible to them. Taking advantage of these sage resources, leaders can fully access for the organization and for themselves the utility of the wisdom, insight, and history of those in the organization who have much to share.

Often, a part of this scenario is the need to formally access and provide continu-ity to use of clinical and management leaders who have much of value to share. Sometimes decisions lacking sage information could lead to organizational chal-lenge or failure. As consultants, we often communicate with more mature staff regarding long-term implications of a particular current crisis or challenge in a system. Often, what we have found is that the current critical issue has a direct or implied relationship to a continuum of decisions and actions predicated on a set of assumptions that could have been better informed had the key stakeholders been a part of the decision. Through the consultant's lens, when leadership uses a succession or leadership handoff system that provides the right information, tools, and insights, many challenges and possible errors in leadership insight and strategy can be easily avoided.

The trajectory of our experiences gives us information with regard to how complex systems work and represents the substance of our development. Along with our learning, our experience provides the platform for translating what we know and what we do in a way that has an impact on our own lives and on other people's lives and experiences. At the same time, the experience and skills of colleagues and others that are significant in our lives have as much an impact on our development and growth, and those people do their part in influencing the course of our lives and the people we become. In our personal life journeys, there is a sort of developmental dance among our learning, our experiences, insights gained from others, and the relationships we share with people with whom we intersect (Patton, Zalon, & Ludwick, 2015). Each of these influences and the sum of them link within our persona to create a unique and individual life lens and insight related to our world and how we have lived in it.

O---▶

"I am not a teacher, but an awakener."

–Robert Frost

One of the joys of this life journey is the increased knowledge, insight, and skill we develop as we aggregate experiences and learning relationships. If we have had an open attitude in all these arenas, we have been available to the opportunities to deepen our insights and understandings and broaden our awareness in a way that helps us develop expertise that advances our talent as professionals. One of the urges this dynamic generates is the desire to share and to extend these insights and talents in a way that benefits others who are also eager for learning and personal development. This desire to share knowledge and skill is an outgrowth of our own openness and availability to learning and personal development. Those individuals who understand this dynamic also recognize that embedded in it is the give-and-take reflected in the interaction of all who share a commitment to growing, learning, and deepening their knowledge and understanding.

For the professional, their community of practice recognizes and affirms both the requisite and desire each member has for both personal development and sharing learning for the benefit of the development of the professional community at large. This developmental relationship over the life of the professional is such an important factor in the health and the success of the professional community that it becomes a requisite of membership and obligation of the professional group to the larger community that the group serves. Embedded deep within the ethos of the profession lies the obligation for relevance and the advancement of practice. For the professional, this obligation means demonstrating a personal commitment to continual self-development as well as a generative obligation to share that development and wisdom with the larger professional community.

LIFE JOURNEY: MENTORSHIP AND SUCCESSION

Over the life of a professional, a continuing and dynamic obligation for personal growth and development and for sharing with peers becomes an obligation that effectively translates into mentorship and succession. Traditionally, as a professional grows, matures, and moves into the senior ranks of his or her professional work group, the professional's learning and experience transforms from personal growth and development toward a general expectation for imparting wisdom, sharing experiences, and generating insights toward influencing, informing, and developing the younger professional (Swanwick & McKimm, 2011). This expectation for sharing wisdom, of course, operates in concert with the wise individual's own desire to communicate and share what has been learned, experienced, and developed into exceptional skill or talent.

Frequently at this stage of maturation we hear these professionals addressed as individuals who are informed, politically astute, knowledgeable, wise, or "at the top of their game." We expect that because of this acknowledgment, these individuals have important things to impart or demonstrate to those at earlier stages of their developmental journeys. Whether formal or informal, this form of mentorship is an expectation of the relationship of the sage or wise person with the younger or less developed in the learning community. Throughout the history of humankind, in a variety of cultures, this mentorship and succession role is described as having a great place in the life of a culture, and both are imbued with the greatest respect and value (Burton-Jones & Spender, 2011).

○---▶

"The mind is not a vessel to be filled, but a fire to be kindled."
–Plutarch

MENTORSHIP AND SUCCESSION

Although there is certainly an implied and an expected understanding that the experienced and skilled individuals in our profession are leaders and mentors in their practice, it is often not formalized into a design for action or a considered approach to utilizing and developing the products of wisdom, knowledge, and skill in a way that positively informs and benefits the individual, health agency, and the community of practice. More often than not, this important role of mentorship and succession is left to the individual sages to determine how much they are willing to communicate and share of what they have gained over the life of their careers. Rather than making mentorship and succession a normative expectation and part of the sage's practice, it remains more option and opportunity than obligation and requisite.

There is increasing—but controversial—discussion as to whether a formal construct of work should include the opportunity for the wise and experienced to play a formal mentorship role that helps to deepen insight and develop practice wisdom in peers and novice practitioners. Much of the controversy centers on the premise that the organization has provided opportunities and a vehicle for the expert to develop experience, skill, and wisdom. It is assumed by these thinkers that a part of the return on the system's investment is this individual's obligation to provide a quid pro quo to the organization by giving back to others through insights gained in the opportunities for growth and success provided by the organization (Raes, Decuyper, & Lismont, 2013). A number of mechanisms has been suggested by these authors for this transfer of wisdom to become a more formalized part of the work of the organization and the profession:

- Design and implement a formal mentorship/succession program where mentors are identified and developed into the mentorship role in a way that enhances their skills related to articulating insight, communicating experience, generating value, and developing mentoring and communication skills.

- Create opportunities for narration and storytelling through regular professional community programs or events. At these formal gatherings, sages and mentors with particular knowledge and skill sets would share learning, experiences, and insights related to their area of leadership and practice in a highly interactive format designed to help facilitate translation and application.

- Provide opportunities for sages or mentors to document through journal writing or personal articles those elements or components of their learning journey, experiences, insights, and wisdom garnered from their leadership/practice experiences. While these journals or articles are meant to provide a personal record for the individual mentor, they can be shared in mentorship sessions, as organizational memoirs (in libraries or historical references), or written as published documents available to the public at large.

- Support opportunities for the sage or mentor to videotape insights through the use of interviews, panels, demonstrations, or presentations from which an archive can be created for users to access and use at their convenience.

- Hold live, online, national or international, moderated sessions for the sage or mentor to share and interact with the larger professional or service community. Construct the sessions in a way that audience members can access wisdom and insight and engage with the sage or mentor in a live question-and-answer portion that emphasizes the relevance and viability to contemporary and future leadership or practice.

These examples are a small sample of the opportunities for general mentorship and sage sharing. They demonstrate mechanisms for formalizing and structuring both the value of mentoring and sharing and the utility of that information in informing and advancing the skills and practices of the larger practice community. Doing so creates both an opportunity and an expectation that such mentoring and succession planning is an ongoing and operating part of the life of the profession in generating knowledge, advancing practice, valuing expertise, and generating new insights.

"True education does not consist merely in the acquiring of a few facts of science, history, literature, or art, but in the development of character."
–David O. McKay

MENTORING AND PROFESSIONAL DEVELOPMENT

Although there is clearly an obligation and opportunity for the sharing of experiences, knowledge, and wisdom gained over a lifetime of career experiences, there's also a personal obligation for all leaders for mentorship and succession (Brockbank & McGill, 2012). In a variety of arenas, the contemporary need for leadership in practice development of individuals is widely apparent. The need, indeed requisite, for creating formal mechanisms of mentorship in light of succession generates from a variety of particular and important demands:

- *Demand to engage younger nurses in leadership*

  There is a paucity of willing and able emergent leaders seeking to engage in the accelerating and complicating demands of contemporary leadership roles in highly complex and transforming healthcare systems. This challenge has reached a critical condition in healthcare. Whether due to the overwhelmingly negative image generated by the apparent stressors and burdens of current leadership, or the accelerating complexity, time demands, and challenges of current leadership roles, there is decreasing interest in assuming these roles among younger members of the professional community. As a result, there is a rapidly increasing need for experienced and talented contemporary leaders to generate an image and capacity for both modeling and engaging professionals with the potential for leadership. The need to translate the role in a way that creates perceptions of excitement, possibility, contribution, and unlimited potential for impact is overwhelming in the current work environment.

- *Demand for leaders to adapt and exemplify the emerging model of healthcare delivery*

  Contemporary healthcare system transformation opportunities and challenges create a demand for new kinds of practice leaders who are able to value past practices but are equally capable of engaging new roles and practices that are as yet undefined. The emerging model for healthcare delivery that emphasizes value over volume, mobility over fixed services, digital facility beyond process orientation, and relational integration over vertical hierarchy calls for a new kind of clinical and practice leadership. Understanding the architecture, structures, and dynamics of the emerging value-based and accountability-driven health system with the capacity to translate these realities into contemporary practice requires unique leadership gifts and talents. Redefining these and role modeling the capacity to adapt is a major obligation of the contemporary leadership mentor.

- *Demand to fulfill the role and contribution expectations of younger nurses*

  Well-prepared novice nurses and other health professionals are now entering the profession with a higher level of expectation regarding role and impact. Due to the past decade of faculty shortages, the opportunity to select the very best and brightest women and men into the profession has accelerated dramatically. However, along with the opportunity for exceptional intellectual talent has come an associated expectation that these gifts will be embraced, exercise the full extent of one's capacity, and be positively expressed by professional colleagues in practice. This expectation has been generally poorly addressed, leaving new graduates in a frustrated state of flux and causing a good percentage of them to leave the institutional practice environment within 2 years of graduation. Those new practitioners who persevere frequently go on to graduate schools for advanced degrees, believing they will achieve a higher level of satisfaction in more independent practice roles. Others leave the profession completely. There is obviously an increasing need to alter these experiences and perceptions to keep these gifted new professionals in the practice setting and provide them ample opportunity for rich experiences, meaningful relationships, and opportunities to grow and develop into the clinical leaders that have the potential to grow into successful leadership roles.

- *Demand to assess and identify potential practice leaders as early as possible*

  Assessment and identification of potential new practice leaders needs to occur at the earliest point of access in their professional careers. Existing experienced leaders need to have the talent for assessing for potential and identifying individuals who demonstrate aptitude for leadership. Meaningful and important relationships between novice and mentor have been demonstrated as a critical and useful tool in early engagement of leadership capacity. Through the establishment of these relationships and interactions, a trajectory of leadership skill development is established. The potential for engaging and embracing future leadership roles is accelerated through this mentorship process and the formal components of the longer-term program, and new leaders can develop in an environment of encouragement and develop their mentorship relationship in a safe space for leadership risk-taking. For the existing contemporary leader, this model provides an opportunity for succession leadership development and offers an arena where his or her learned gifts have an opportunity to affect the development of others.

Much has been gained by the individual leader over the long course of her or his leadership journey. These leaders have developed significant and important insights, experiences, and capacity, which results in a large armamentarium of insights and skills that have real utility and value. Imagine how disappointing it is when such important insights and skills are developed but remain essentially locked inside the experienced leader. Here, within the life of the mature leader, is a full range of unique and important attributes, characteristics, and practices that have significance and value when perceived through the lens of the emergent leader (see the following feature). This new leader, perhaps experienced and well educated in the practice arena, may be pregnant with leadership possibility yet is an empty vessel with regard to experience, knowledge, and skill. Through the intersection of the relationship between these two professionals, the value-based partnership should be formally constructed and not left either to neglect or chance, as often occurs in many organizations. Such elements and characteristics of leadership succession are essential to the future viability of the health system and of those who will lead it.

THE DIFFERENCE PERSONAL MENTORING MAKES

Very early in my career, I was given the opportunity to be a protégé and mentee of Irma E. Goertzen, MN, RN, who was assistant administrator of patient services at Providence Medical Center in Seattle, Washington. She recognized early signs of my potential leadership abilities and encouraged me to construct a plan that would develop those skills. At that time I was an associate degree nurse who had no clear plans of continuing my education. Irma promoted me to a shift manager role and established regular meeting times with me to talk about my under-addressed career development plan.

With her wisdom, insight, and care, I was able to develop an education and leadership development trajectory that would help prepare me for the possibility of growing and expanding my leadership potential. Irma helped me develop flexibility in my schedule to accommodate learning in my BSN program, served as my advocate and provided recommendations for entry into the master's program, and provided me experiential opportunity through a leadership growth trajectory at the medical center while I was still learning. All through this time, she continued regular and formal mentoring sessions that helped me with both personal and role leadership development through the use of job opportunities and challenges in the workplace. She drew from her own experience, wisdom, and political insight to help me deal with interprofessional and disciplinary processes that helped me mature in my growing and transitioning leadership role. To her credit, and her personal commitment to growing me in the profession, she even suggested when she thought it was time I leave the organization and move into a more significant leadership role, which I did.

I continued to depend on Irma's sage and wise counsel throughout the course of my leadership career. I cannot count the times I drew on her advice and wisdom in moments of challenge and crises. In addition, her enthusiasm for the profession, the significance of the role of the nurse, and her commitment to me and to the person of the nurse in me generated a continuing personal joy and zest for our profession and the opportunities it provided to make a difference in the world.

Irma demonstrated her own leadership in succession planning by nurturing me where I was planted and handing off to me the skills and insights learned in her lifetime of leadership. She mentored me through my developmental transitions and maturation as I struggled to meet the challenges of my leadership trajectory. To this day, when I envision the image of my leadership ideal, it is Irma's face I see.

Following are the five key things that I learned from Irma Goertzen that have informed my leadership and my rules of mentorship over the course of my career:

1. Begin early with leadership development. Discern and capture the potential for leadership in others as soon you observe it and help them begin their leadership trajectory while they are still new and fresh in the role.

2. Mentorship is primarily about relationships and caring. There must be a genuine sense of fondness and connection between mentor and mentee that facilitates the development of real personal communion at a level of communication that engages both the spirit and the potential of the leader within.

3. Regular interaction, communication, and meeting times are important to establishing the discipline of mentorship and leadership development. It takes time to develop and mature the leader within and involves not only conversation in the passage of essential information and learning, but also identification, role modeling, and demonstration of the lessons learned on the leader's journey.

4. Experiment and conduct small tests of application. Leadership is a learned skill. Most of that learning comes from application and practice. Repeated efforts followed by evaluation and recalibration are critical to developing and refining leadership capacity and skill. My mentor provided fresh insight with regard to testing out application, but I still had to do the work and take the risks.

5. Leadership development is a journey rather than an event. There is no sprinting to the front of the leadership line. There is only perseverance and hard slogging through each day of challenge, some frustration, and small measures of success. Leadership excellence grows over time and its excellence in expression is a discovery. I learned to take time to celebrate small successes and to share my successes with others. Thus, I developed my own mentorship skills and began to have meaningful learning to give to others.

—Tim Porter-O'Grady, DM, EdD, ScD(h), APRN, FAAN, FACCWS

HANDOFF AND SUCCESSION

Succession should not be an incidental or accidental event in any organization. The ability to prepare for the future and to assure that future generations have what they need to thrive and succeed in a highly transforming environment should never be optional if the organization is to thrive. Nursing experts and leaders have much to offer new nurses growing into roles with increasing responsibility. They can be both informed and comforted from the insights gained from practice and leadership sages that have been through it all before. Even if the context and the environment continue to shift away from traditional landscapes of practice, the skills of learning, adaptation, and accommodation and the personal struggles related to handling challenges can be exceptionally useful to new nurses.

The need for a connection between experienced and competent leaders in an organization and emergent members of that same organization is not really optional in any successful system. However, not leaving such matters to chance means the organization takes a serious and formal approach to the issue of succession, and it's the organization leaders who see succession as a personal obligation of their leadership roles and as a fundamental expression of the leadership capacity (Piper, 2012). If leaders are competent and impactful and it makes a difference in the lives of people and organizations, the leaders have much to contribute in sharing those experiences with others who are just beginning their leadership careers.

Failure to share these contributions does not serve the organization, the sage leader, or the emergent leader (whether clinical or managerial), who will hold many of those leadership roles in the future. In order to understand why, you need only to ask the question, "How many experiences of marginal clinical or management leadership value could have been bypassed or completely avoided had good leadership mentorship and insight been shared in succession with emerging leaders before they assumed roles where those same issues were confronted?" Issues related to staffing and scheduling, conflict management, vagaries of wide-ranging personality characteristics, personal uncertainties related to new clinical practices, and interactional and relational challenges with colleagues, patients, and families could all be better handled with tools gained from those sages and experienced nurses who now handle such issues with comfort and skill.

Real and effective professional handoffs in succession require concerted attention to the following specific realities:

- *Our recognition of the value and significance of our experience and insight*

  There must be a sense of self-value and of legitimacy with regard to the substance of what individuals have to hand off. If we don't have a firm belief that we have something of inherent value that rises to the significance of transferability, it is equally difficult to see any reason to share it. This personal sense of value informs both the understanding of the importance of our experience or wisdom and how the vision of the capacity translates into a value worth sharing. Self-worth and the importance of our learning and experience are an important first step in recognizing the meaning and transferability of personal wisdom and experience. How much valuable insight and skill are lost to the ages because the individual whose life was committed to honing and refining expertise never felt the worth of it enough to recognize the need to share and transfer it? This failure to see the value of personal wisdom and experience is especially true for nurses who, through a torturous history of oppression and second-class status, received scant public acknowledgment of their impact and value. Most nurses in the discipline never develop the first-line professional identity where the work of what is gained over a lifetime of learning is expected to be on public display as it is in other disciplines (medicine, law, architecture, engineering, and so on).

• *Organizational commitment to the continuity of knowledge and competency handoffs*

Organizations must recognize that knowledge and competency handoffs are essential to the continuity and sustainability of their trajectory toward continuing success. Long-thriving organizations have a reputation for honoring contribution and building links between generations such that contributions continue over the long term. Organizations that demonstrate strong leadership and an ability to succeed repeatedly over generations exemplify a well-developed continuum of leadership growth, mentorship, internal opportunities for progression, and succession. Each of these frames of reference demonstrates the organization's capability to inculcate the dynamic of handing off wisdom, expertise, and leadership along an unbroken continuum that assures consistency and continuity over the life of the organization. Hospitals and health systems have not done as well with these definitive organs of continuity, often leaving a significant amount of personal insight and experience on the doorsteps of resignation, retirement, or other turnover. Indeed, the often inexorable ease of onboarding and offboarding nurses and other knowledge resources has served to diminish both the value and exercise of knowledge management, handoffs, and the continuity of professional growth and advancement in many health systems. As a result we continue to struggle with issues of competence, quality, sustainable impact, and risk. The simple inclusion of a systematic approach to development, advancement, succession, and handoffs in the health system would go far to remedy these challenges.

- *The significance and strength of the mentor–mentee bond*

Establishment of a sound professional relationship is a cornerstone of the mentorship characterized by the handoff of wisdom and good succession strategies. Societies in which wisdom and age are valued and the expectation is that wisdom is generously shared have a meaningful and generative interaction between generations. In the United States, where social relationships and interaction are more fast-paced and that which is new, different, and emergent has superordinate value, it is much more difficult to establish sound communication linkages between generations. As a result, in many organizations, leaders are sentenced to repetitiveness, and waste is a constant element in strategy, decision-making, and action. How many strategies, decisions, or undertakings that failed could have been avoided if experience with those same conditions and circumstances in the past had been drawn upon to influence the kind and quality of subsequent decisions?

Just because contemporary circumstances may be altered by a transforming environment does not mean that every new occurrence is devoid of historical content. Human experience, reflection, and discernment from previous transactions, iterations, or transformations can serve to inform meaning, reflection, and insight in a way that provides context for current contemporary circumstances. When we value the "discipline of the wisdom of time," we are provided with a more cautious and wise methodology for translating environmental impact, contextual influences, and circumstances that guide response and action to the demand for meaningful change and growth. In leadership, this is especially important. The mentor–mentee interaction provides more than an opportunity for wisdom that assures a continuity of growth; it also builds on previously gained insights that serve as the information foundation for the emerging leader. Furthermore, it saves this person from having to begin his or her leadership from "ground-zero" and being doomed to repeat errors of the past. Significance or "tightness" of the relationship between mentor and mentee can guarantee the upward trajectory of leadership growth, assuring that it endures to expand and build on previously gained discernment and wisdom.

Succession structures and processes inside a system and associated with leadership create the potential to sift through history, experience, and insight to select the best each of these has to offer and apply it to the organization and its leaders. The development of a strong and formalized mentorship, handoff, and succession approach creates a dynamic inside the system that sees growth and excellence as a template from which the organization measures success. By using and applying the wisdom, learning, knowledge, and insights gained from mature and experienced members in the organization, the organization can lay a new foundation or "floor" for leadership and work practices. Further improvements and enhancements in practices and behaviors can build from that new floor of wisdom and learning, continually accelerating the trajectory of growth, improvement, and enhancement in a way that assures the organization is able to continually raise the bar. When the gems that are gained from the contribution of mature members of the organization are used, the system is better positioned to compete and to thrive in an ever-shifting marketplace. This systematic and continuous approach to organizational lifelong learning creates a net aggregated benefit for the organization.

In addition, this formalized infrastructure of valuing knowledge, insight, and experience and incorporating it into the data set for strategy, decision-making, and initiatives gives the organization a leg up on its competition with an internal operating structure that makes mentoring and handing off knowledge a part of its way of doing business. In such a system, expectations abound at every level of the structure: Mature, experienced, wise sages have a medium for communicating the value of their history in an organization that is receptive to it; emerging clinical and management leaders are identified and accessed in a way that associates them with mentors and advisors who can refine and develop their talents to a higher degree of sophistication and value; the system is a methodology and a framework for including the insight and wisdom of its sages in its environmental scanning, strategic processes, and tactical decisions. Within the context of such a system, several values set it apart from the ordinary:

- A real valuing of the wisdom and insight of its sages

- A belief in the need to access the insights and wisdom of the sage in a way that affects the organization and its people

- A dynamic and continuous mentor–mentee relationship that is structured as a centerpiece of the organization's leadership growth and development function

- A systematic and organized structure and process within the organization assuring the valuing of the sages, the utility of their contributions, the transition of their skills, and the effectiveness of their handoffs are inculcated within the organization's way of doing business

In this way, both person and system demonstrate how intensely the contribution of the mature and wise leaders is valued. Here an organized system of communication provides mechanisms for assuring that wisdom is not lost. This communication support system assures that those who are emerging into the roles of clinical and management leadership have access to that learning and can themselves do their part in developing and expanding the wisdom that others will one day draw upon to the benefit of those who will continue to create our future (Brown, 2014).

PERSONAL REFLECTIONS

Tim and I have worked hard to reflect these principles and beliefs in our partnership over the past 20 years. Early in our partnership we realized that we had admiration and respect for each other's areas of expertise and passion for excellence. Tim is the broader, deeper thinker and futurist, whereas I am the translator of complex topics and the operational expert. In light of our different but complementary strengths, our respect for each other's work has been without question or exception.

The nature of our writing deserves special mention. We have written books and articles together over the course of our partnership that reflect our regard for each other's content. As previously noted, during our retreat we try to determine what we will write in the coming year. We have never edited each other's work and have provided feedback only on the overall content and value of the content to our readers. We have left the grammatical editing to our editors. As we were writing the first edition of *Quantum Leadership*, I experienced a horrible moment of panic. The editor had *edited* my chapters, and there were more red marks on the pages than black ink! I was horrified at my lack of writing expertise and called Tim to advise him that, because of the significant amount of editing, I probably was not the best person to write with him. He was calm and asked me whether the editors had changed any of the meaning of my content. The answer was no—they actually improved the presentation of the information. He laughed and advised me to let the editors keep their jobs. After all, if they had not put some red on the pages, then they had not been doing their jobs. I continue to stick to the content edits and no longer worry about the red ink. This experience in my writing journey can encourage other novice authors to remain engaged in sharing the content of their expertise and, when necessary, rely on expert editors to do their work as well.

Worth sharing is that we have also learned that our trust in each other and ability to predict what each of us is thinking have increased dramatically. From the mentorship perspective, we have recognized the importance of patience, consistency, and openness with each other. With each passing year, we take time at retreats to validate our uniqueness, to affirm that we are not speaking for each other, and to always validate the accuracy of what we are presenting. The openness and transparency of our relationship cannot be underestimated as the foundation of our success. This very special dance between colleagues suggests a continuing effort at developing the fluidity that results in being available for opportunities that might emerge, discussing the implications, and never being afraid of the future.

PERSONAL APPLICATION

The following questions are designed to help you reflect on the knowledge and wisdom you have gained over your career and to facilitate the successful transfer of this knowledge and wisdom to those nurse leaders who, like you, have devoted their life's work to their patients and to the nursing profession.

1. Handing off between generations is a fundamental obligation of professional relations and mentorship. It assures the continuity of learning, honors the past, and grounds the future.

   - As you review your own experience, describe either an opportunity or an occurrence where the transfer of nursing knowledge occurred from a mentor or an expert directly to you.

   - What example from your own life experience demonstrates your role in handing off knowledge or experience to a new nurse?

   - As you view your own life experiences, what predominant two or three skills, insights, or pieces of knowledge do you now feel have the most value to transfer to others?

2. Keeping knowledge and experiences alive from one generation to the next is an important part of establishing continuity of learning that reflects both evidence and standards of practice.

   - Describe ways where you and your peers use the insight and experience practitioners use in assessing and making judgments about foundations and standards of practice.

   - What is the role that professional experience plays in establishing evidence-based foundations for practice?

   - Select an example from your own history where your practice experience and advice were used to evaluate a standard or best practice.

- How often have you seen yourself as an expert and from that perspective have been willing to share and contribute insights related to your experience and standards of practice?

3. This chapter discusses your profession as a part of your life's journey. For a professional, the profession becomes a part of one's person.

    - In what ways have you and do you demonstrate to others how integral your connection to the profession is to your life's journey?
    - What challenges have you confronted with others in the profession that have tested your commitment to the profession?
    - What are some ways you can help new professionals embrace their professional journey and develop tools to remain faithful to this commitment?
    - What is your strategy for dealing with others who have negative things to say about nursing and discourage others, and how can you pass that on to new nurses who will confront the same issues?

4. Attitude toward continuous and dynamic change in nursing and healthcare is critical to how that change will take form and move persons and organizations to improve health services in each generation.

    - What is your own attitude to the constancy of change and how has that been represented in your own behavior and response to the demands of change?
    - What sage advice would you give new nurses with regard to healthcare change and the insights they may need to embrace and engage in their practice?
    - When a change needs to be refined or scrapped because it is not working, how have you participated in making that adjustment and positively modeled that engagement for others?

5. A formal mentorship and handoff program in the nursing organization is necessary to validate the value of practice and leadership succession between generations of nurses.

- Do you have a role to play in developing a formal approach to mentorship and transition that values the opportunity to hand off wisdom and skills between the generations?

- Are you open to the new learning and insights you can gain from younger generations and incorporating their new insights into your own practice life?

- Is it safe in your organization for new nurses to speak out and to be heard when their insights run counter to the prevailing view?

- How do you advocate for next-generation nurses in a way that creates a sense of belonging, involvement, and ownership for them in the life of your practice community?

LOOKING FORWARD

There is no doubt that the collective wisdom of those people who are dedicated to making a difference can truly move mountains and achieve lofty goals. But this doesn't occur without a considerable level of intention. In this chapter we attempted to communicate as specifically and clearly as possible that the role of the sage and the wisdom he or she represents is critical to successful transition, handing off, and succession. The experienced and wise administrative or practice leader has two obligations: provide a systematic and organized mechanism for the compilation, transfer, and utility of wisdom and experience in a way that has meaning and value for new and emerging nurses; and demonstrate both willingness and capacity to act as wise sage and mentor to others in a dynamic, interactive, and engaging relationship that provides a bridge between wisdom and the emergent and energetic learning capacity of new nurses. Through this partnership between a structure for mentorship and succession and the practices and action of mentorship and handing off, the continuum of growing, learning, becoming, experiencing, and gaining wisdom becomes a seamless dynamic between generations of nurses committed to continuing to act in the best interest of those they serve.

"All the world's a stage, and All the men and women merely players: They have their exits and their entrances; And one man in his time plays many parts, His acts begin seven ages."

—William Shakespeare

2

PREPARATION FOR KNOWLEDGE & WISDOM TRANSFER

MARY LOCKHART, PHD, MS
DOROTHY SISNEROS, MS, MBA, FAACVPR

CHAPTER OBJECTIVES

Describe the three different types of transitions that necessitate attention to knowledge management, and ways to address handoffs for each.

Provide guidelines for prioritizing content areas for knowledge transfer.

Describe approaches for "letting go" and ways to prepare oneself and others for transition.

Understand the "how" and the "what" that guide effective knowledge transfer, as well as how generational preferences may inform effective approaches.

This chapter focuses on improving our preparedness for work transitions that will benefit from a handoff of knowledge and wisdom. To guide you toward this level of preparedness, we provide the following fundamental questions for you to consider and explore:

- How do we let go when it's time? How can we help others let go?

- Who (besides us) cares about our work?

- How do we determine what the next generation or successor needs?

- What things should we not worry about passing on?

- Is it possible to quantify knowledge for a handoff?

To enrich the responses, we interviewed five accomplished healthcare professionals to share their experiences and recommendations. These foundational questions, which we also asked our interviewees, may be ones we intuitively (and sometimes unconsciously) ask ourselves, with hopes that this chapter will give them voice.

A CRITICAL NEED FOR KNOWLEDGE TRANSFER

During a recent healthcare experience, I became focused on the ease with which caregivers shared and received information about my history and my current condition. They used the electronic medical record (EMR) and other technology to track day-to-day, week-to-week, and month-to-month changes in my status. I realized that these nurses and other caregivers had mastered the handoff of information and knowledge, and the dynamic nature of my situation required them to share seamlessly. The seamless handoffs gave me confidence that my treatment was supported by documentation and subjective reports about my progress with others on the team.

Just like the members of my healthcare team, leaders are tasked with sharing information with colleagues that will provide the background and context for decision-making and ensure a productive workplace. However, our competency in effectively handing off knowledge to new leaders is much more challenged (as this chapter illustrates), and the identification of best practices to address today's challenges is clearly still evolving. As healthcare transformation occurs at a more rapid pace than any time in history, the ability to transfer essential knowledge has become more critical, and it affects patient care on a more global scale.

Research on knowledge management and knowledge transfer is relatively new, as both fields began to receive focused attention in the early 1990s. The questions of *what* information to leave and *to whom* to leave it continue to challenge leaders and organizations worldwide. Both areas have received even more focused attention, given the pending departure of the baby boomer generation from the workforce, the potential for large knowledge drains, and the change in the current workforce. Nearly 30% of the healthcare workforce is 55 or older (Society for Human Resource Management [SHRM], 2014). We know that the large numbers who comprise the baby boomer generation are at or nearing retirement age. If the nearly 70% of leaders within this group retire in the next few years, organizations will face the loss of leadership, skills/knowledge, and relationships developed over years. If we do not put in place processes to transfer knowledge from these individuals, this knowledge leaves when the leader exits. This reality is compounded by the job-hopping tendencies of the millennial generation and will result in a dramatic impact on business productivity and the ability to compete in today's environment (McGraw, 2013).

Interestingly, the SHRM study also found that fewer than one-third of all organizations considered the loss of older talent as a crisis or a significant problem in their industry, and 36% indicated that they were preparing for the expected loss of older workers. Only 4% of organizations claim to have a strategy in place to retain older workers. However, more than 54% of respondents indicated that they are focused on cross-training programs aimed at transferring knowledge from older workers via shadowing, cross-training, mentoring programs, and the development of succession plans. These statistics seem to suggest that many healthcare organizations are recognizing that leader successions are coming, and they may be preparing for, but are not particularly concerned with, the loss of seasoned leaders or the wisdom they might bring to this discussion.

This leaves us to wonder whether organizations have a clear understanding of the sheer numbers that can retire or the fact that there are many other competing priorities. Regardless, failure to address and plan for this reality will add to the knowledge drain. With healthcare CEO turnover rates at their highest level in history—at more than 20% in 2013 (Larkin, 2015)—and the changing demands on leaders in healthcare, the landscape is ripe for a plan on how to manage the transitions in a thoughtful manner. The nursing profession needs new leadership skills to navigate the changes, and these nurse leaders must be change champions who focus on how data informs all decisions. Nurses can make excellent senior leaders because of their management and clinical expertise. Skills of the past may not serve the leadership needs of the future at all levels of the organization. When using retiring leaders to mentor new leaders, this potential limitation will need to be considered to ensure effective transition planning.

TECHNOLOGY AS A CONDUIT FOR KNOWLEDGE TRANSFER

Technology is being used to gather, reproduce, and transfer knowledge, and the number of IT firms specializing in this area has exploded. There is a belief that if we gather, store, and reproduce knowledge, it has been transferred. Of course, we know this is not the case, and this belief is illusory. Reliance on technology may appear to solve the problem, as you can upload data, documents, forms, facts, and other explicit information to the cloud or other storage system, but the who, why, how, when (tacit information), and the knowledge that comes from valued relationships cannot be completely captured. The nuances of how decisions were made or the brainstorming and process used to make critical or everyday decisions cannot be uploaded.

PERSONAL KNOWLEDGE MANAGEMENT

As critical tacit and explicit knowledge is identified, the challenge of how, what, to whom, and where to transfer knowledge is complicated by the huge numbers of workers expected to leave the workforce in the upcoming years. We must also consider that in addition to organizational knowledge, personal knowledge management is in play and needs to be addressed. This section explores three different types of knowledge management concerns—planned transitions, transitions or departures, and unplanned transitions—and provides tips on how to thoughtfully and effectively address each concern to minimize the impact of each on the individual, workplace, and workforce.

PLANNED TRANSITIONS

Employees who anticipate and plan for a departure (usually retirement) are provided with a unique opportunity for the intentional and methodical transfer of knowledge once a successor has been identified.

Large companies such as American Express and Kaiser have considered the impact of projected retirements of seasoned and experienced leaders. They have succession plans in place to address this expected disruption. What to hand off and what to keep is planned, methodical, and organized. Upcoming leaders are identified and groomed in anticipation of the departure of a key leader. In healthcare, however, succession planning is fairly new, not standard, and has not reached all levels of the organization.

TRANSITIONS OR DEPARTURES

Employees who voluntarily terminate their employment and move to another organization have the potential to cause a major disruption in short-term and long-term projects. Unless the organization has identified a successor for a handoff, the usual 2- to 4-week period of transition may result in a disorderly transfer of knowledge or a situation in which the employees leave the organization without the opportunity to hand off their knowledge at all; they walk out the door with important, and sometimes critical, knowledge, including what has been called "political wisdom." Finally, the information may need to be transferred to several individuals, and the "whole" is lost.

Deb K.,* an experienced healthcare quality and business leader, shared her experience in transitioning from a job and the process used:

> *The job I was doing needed to be farmed out to five different*
> *people over the course of 3 months, with responsibility for IT,*
> *finance, patient care, quality, and ongoing administration*
> *going to different people. It wasn't too difficult to figure out*
> *what the priorities were or who these people would be (I had*

---

*Deb K. has been a healthcare leader in the areas of clinical quality and business integration for more than 30 years.

worked with them), though they had to have more than ex-
pertise—they had to be open to growing and learning more
to meet the new needs of the organization that would evolve.
The process involved orienting each one of them to their tasks
in a 3-month period of time, providing them with enough
skill, knowledge, tools, and background (politics, etc.) as
possible.

The key is to understand that old rules and assumptions may not apply when new leaders take ownership. What one person sees as important and critical may not be on the radar for the successor. When planning time is shortened, what to hand off and what to keep can be haphazard, disjointed, and insufficient.

UNPLANNED TRANSITIONS

Employees who are terminated or die suddenly leave a void that cannot be filled. In the case of the employee who is terminated, the usual "walk them out the door" situation leaves the organization with huge gaps in workflow. Relationships are damaged even if the employee termination was warranted. There is a realization that remaining employees and teams have to pick up the extra workload, start over, or depend on others to piece together information and knowledge without the ability to call and ask questions—or, in some cases, to find out what happened. For those organizations that have a sudden death, the transition is complicated by the unexpected departure and grieving for the leader. The organization must reassess its direction, recommit, or start over. Unless a formal succession planning process was in place, the organization may struggle with continuation of the work. In some cases, chaos and jockeying for power may occur.

SMOOTHLY PASSING THE BATON

As a department chair in higher education, I had made the decision to leave my organization after 12 years of building a solid team and department. I had the conversation with administration. Because of the nature of how leaders are selected in higher education, the department was able to identify my successor, and we set about methodically transferring my knowledge, experience, and relationships to the successor. Over the course of the year, the successor shadowed me in critical meetings, attended meetings in my place, led department meetings, and participated in every aspect of the role. In the final semester prior to my departure, I moved out of my office, and the successor became the department chairperson and assumed all duties of the role. I was able to be there for support while redirecting others to go to her for all decisions. When it was time to leave, I walked out knowing that our legacy would continue, and after 12 years, she remains in the role as a respected leader. The key here is that we can and should take the time to provide the opportunity for both parties to assume new roles and for both parties to graciously accept the changes that were planned and executed with the team involved.

—Dorothy Sisneros, MS, MBA, FAACVPR

"People in their handlings of affairs often fail when they are about to succeed. If one remains as careful at the end as he was at the beginning, there will be no failure."

—Lao-Tzu

Now that you understand the types of personal knowledge management, the following sections explore questions you may want to consider as you plan for—or experience—work transitions and handoffs to others.

HOW TO LET GO

After the transition decision has been made (by you and/or others), "letting go" in a thoughtful way can help you—and others—envision the change and prepare to move forward. Needless to say, this task is easier when it's *your* decision to leave an organization, and you have sufficient time to think about how you want to do this. For instance, Deb K. thought a lot about her life priorities before making the decision to move to a position that allowed her more freedom: "I realized that much of my life had been about taking care of others—I wanted to make room for me and had the financial resources to make it possible." When the way in which the job transition happened was not planned or was painful, however, letting go can take years (often beyond the period of employment with that organization). Susan B.,[*] a seasoned nurse and CEO, while enjoying her financial and time freedom, continues to make peace with unknowns and what to do next. Alice S.,[**] an experienced nurse practitioner, found that although she loved the patients, the team, and the work, her current employment situation was unhealthy and it was time to move to something new.

William Bridges, author of *Managing Transitions* (2009), provides a number of helpful tips and guidance for constructive ways on how to consider your transition and the impact it will have on others:

- *Share details about the transition.*

  Describe the change in as much detail as you can. Tell others what you know when you know it (for example, "You will have a new boss," or, "Our reorganization will happen in stages, and

---

[*]Susan B. is a seasoned nurse who served as a CEO for 12 years at four different organizations.
[**]Alice S. is an experienced nurse practitioner who has managed her own practice and worked with colleagues in several urgent care centers.

you'll have more certainty in about 6 months"). As Laura G.*, an experienced organizational development leader, noted: "It's important to make sure people understand the 'why' behind decisions being made and who they can connect with so they could better understand what would come next for them."

• *Identify the real and potential ripple effects.*

Before you let go completely, consider the secondary changes that your transition will probably cause, and describe what will be different when each change is complete (as best you can). Bridges encourages us to imagine that the change (your transition, others' transitions) is a cue ball rolling across the surface of a pool table. The cue ball hits some balls intentionally and other balls unintentionally. The goal, of course, is to try to foresee as many hits as you can.

One of the author's former bosses, Deb K. (who left the organization as the "pool table" was being set up), helped our team understand the landscape of change in doing an exercise with us she called "Groundhog Day" (named after the famous Bill Murray movie). During the staff meeting, she identified several likely scenarios (each day a new Groundhog Day) and invited the team to discuss the potential impact on them, how we do our work, and the role they may play. Although this exercise did not result in a completely accurate picture of what came to be, this invaluable discussion served to lessen our collective anxiety, prepare the group for change, and to become as informed as we could during the impending transitions.

---

*Laura G. is a seasoned healthcare organizational development leader who worked in a large healthcare system.

- *Acknowledge who and what you are leaving behind.*

When you have identified the chain of cause-and-effect "collisions," think of the people whose familiar way of being will be affected: Who is going to have to let go of something? And what will they be letting go of? (Their peer group? The roles that helped them feel a sense of competence? A relationship with a boss they felt understood them? Their chances for a promotion? Old expectations?) As you think about the collisions, think about what *you* are losing as well (a sense of belonging, competence, confidence, and so on). Ask yourself what is changing for you personally. If you allow yourself to think about this deeply, you will be better prepared to fill in the blanks sincerely for this statement: "I will miss you all, and here's what has made you all special to me: _____." As a nurse practitioner, Alice S. was concerned with the patients she would leave behind, the lives she had impacted, and the hope that they would be in good hands with other providers. For her, it was critical that her patients were left without a gap in care and the confidence that they would be in good hands.

- *Recognize the intangible losses you are experiencing.*

Notice that some losses are not concrete. They are part of the complex interweaving of attitudes, assumptions, and expectations we all hold on to—what Bridges refers to as the things that make us feel "at home in our world." Sometimes the personal losses compel us to accept "incomplete work" on a difficult issue. For instance, a couple of the interviewees spoke about relational barriers, including "unbalanced relationships" that never felt resolved when they left the organization. Examples include circumstances where your values and the organizational values were out of sync or personal relationships with peers that were always strained.

- *Acknowledge the loss others are experiencing openly and honestly.*

Beyond these specific losses, Bridges encourages us to ask if there is something that is over for everyone. Is it a particular chapter in the organization's history? The organization's mission or something the organization stands for? If a change is already underway, you can find out about losses by simply asking people (and yourself) openly. For example, you might ask: "What's different since this change happened?" and "What do you miss?" It is important to acknowledge losses and changes openly, and sympathetically, with staff. This could be as simple as saying, "I'm sorry these changes are upsetting to you. I wish I could make this easier for you. I'm struggling with this as well."

LETTING GO—A PERSONAL JOURNEY

There is only so much knowledge and experience you can transfer, so it's important to prioritize the essentials. As you begin your transition, consider the following:

- Convey the "whys" more than the "hows." Knowing the thinking behind a product, process, or tradition will help the new leader's future decision-making.
- Prepare to feel vulnerable. You may not be used to having to explain or answer questions about your day-to-day decisions and habits. Decide how you want to feel and how you hope others feel about you after you go, and align your behavior accordingly.

- Speak positively of your successor, no matter what you think of the selection. Your direct reports will take their cue from you.

- Don't try to solve all of the problems before you leave. Chances are, your successor was drawn to the job in part because there are problems to solve.

- Refrain from judging the incoming leader as incompetent based on questions or reactions to the way things are done now. Remember that you were new once, too.

- Make a list of your accomplishments in the role, and share that list with your boss and your direct reports. This ensures that you are honored for the things you want to be remembered for, and it helps prevent awkward reinterpretations of your legacy. (It will also help you with your resume for your next job.)

- Give people time and opportunity to express their appreciation before you go. It's important for them to be able to say thank you as part of their process of saying goodbye. You may be surprised at how affirmed you feel. Take that affirmation into whatever you will be doing next.

- Don't make any solo decisions about future events, staffing, or work teams after your successor starts. If the new leader will be obligated to follow through on those decisions, it's only fair that he or she be involved in making them. A partnership mentality helps.

- Decide a specific date when you are no longer going to answer questions from your staff. After that date, consistently redirect questions to the new leader. Offer advice if you feel you can be helpful; avoid getting invested in whether your successor follows your advice. It's not your call anymore.

- In a similar vein, begin handing off routine tasks as soon as possible. The new leader will appreciate being able to contribute right away, and you can focus on completing your larger commitments.

- Ensure the new leader is oriented to the organizational culture and informal roles as well as to meetings and tasks. How do people typically interact? Who is trusted with keys and codes? Who makes the coffee? Organizes birthday lunches? This orientation process may seem trivial, but it goes a long way toward helping the new person feel at home.
- Clear your calendar for your final few days in the office. No matter how long you've been planning the transition, you will still need that time to finish cleaning out paper and computer files. It also allows your mind to bring to the surface those last few critical things you wanted to remember to hand off. Use that time to express your final thank-yous as well.
- Remember that in any organization, nobody is indispensable; the important things will still get done. When it's time to leave, go.

—Laura G. (June 2015)

"One never notices what has been done; one can only see what remains to be done."

—Marie Curie

HOW TO MOVE ON

Whether our transition is planned or not, we all ask ourselves this question and hope (deeply) that we have made a contribution and a difference to others and the organization. Truth be told, however, we may never know the impact we have had.

Sometimes, planned and unplanned transitions may overlap. Susan B., a CEO of a hospital on the East Coast of the United States, was involved in an acquisition and the new owners asked her and other executives to stay as the CEO to assist with the transition. There were promises of financial incentives and the possibility of continuing in the role. She agreed to the planned transition knowing that a new leader would eventually be engaged to carry the hospital forward. Over the ensuing year, she carefully and methodically began the transfer of knowledge to others on the executive team, always sharing the background, rationale, and approach taken to come to the decisions regarding a partnership, relationship, or purchase. All records were updated, and information sharing occurred with the new company leaders.

The successors willingly engaged in the transfer of knowledge so that the legacy and mission would be carried forward. Unfortunately, in the end, when the final deal was sealed, the new leaders "walked her out" and fired the rest of the executive team except for one leader. She left without the opportunity to say goodbye to a team she had led for more than 5 years. All of the strategic preparation was wasted, and her feelings of disregard for the work that had preceded the acquisition were prevalent. It didn't matter to the new leaders as they would move forward without the past. She has not recovered and feels disrespected, used, and like "I was never there" or they just "hit the delete button." Of course, patients continued to be cared for, and the hospital continues to operate.

When the transition is a rapid or unwanted departure, there is an assumption that no one cared about the departing individual and his or her contribution to the organization. In some cases, the way in which some transitions occur is so uncaring that it has the potential to make us question the mission and philosophy of healthcare. We might even think, "People care; organizations don't." Susan B. puts it this way: "Organizations are living entities. They are organic and dynamic, and they pause, adjust, and move on—they have to."

"Educating the mind without educating the heart is no education at all."

–Aristotle

HOW TO IDENTIFY WHAT TO HAND OFF

Whether addressing issues of staff retention, patient safety, complying with regulatory rules, or meeting budget, large demands are being made of professionals in nursing leadership positions today (Sherman, 2013). This reality suggests that handoffs to new leaders will be challenging, particularly when there is a short timeline available to accomplish them. Susan B. shares the following helpful guidelines on determining what new nurse leaders may need:

- Use regulatory requirements, Joint Commission standards, policies and procedures, the organization's mission/vision and values, and the organization's intended direction to guide your decisions.

- Always focus on your patients' needs.

- Consider the knowledge of your successors.

- Share critical information in small pieces and share scenarios with them to convey serious or fragile information.

- Prepare your successors to move from a patient-focused organization to a financially driven organization, sharing with them how they would need to lead in that environment.

- Help new leaders envision themselves in their new roles with different scenarios after you are gone.

The "how to transfer knowledge" question is as important (or more important) than the "what knowledge to transfer" question, particularly in consideration of a cross-generational healthcare workforce. By understanding the values of different generational cohorts, a leader can more effectively translate information and increase the likelihood that the new leader will stay (McGraw, 2013). Boychuk-Duchscher and

Cowin (2004) point out that the four generations of nurses (veterans, baby boomers, Generation X, and millennials) have unique work ethics, different perspectives on work, and distinctly preferred ways of learning, managing, and being managed (see Figure 2.1). Ensuring advancement opportunities and effective coaching can go a long way toward keeping new younger leaders (and employees in general) engaged—and retaining them.

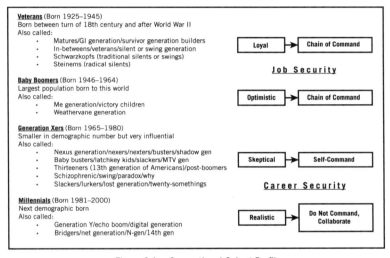

Figure 2.1   Generational Cohort Profile

Younger cohorts "want to be led, not managed" (Kutin, 2012), and this philosophy should begin with the handoff process. The growing demand to address coaching needs requires building the capacity to train and nurture effective coaches and mentors who are leaders, as well as training and nurturing seasoned and/or newer nurses with specific skills. Peg F.,* an ICU and hospice nurse for more than 30 years, shares:

My boss recognized early on that I had a passion, commitment—and talent—for working with patients who

---

*Peg F. is a seasoned RN with more than 30 years of critical care and hospice nursing experience.

were nearing the end of their life (and working with their families). I started to take all of the end-of-life patients. I mentored peers who had an interest and needed help having the "conversation" with patients and their families. Before I knew it, nurses would come back to me and say, "Oh, Peg, you would have been so proud of me."

"Let whoever is in charge keep this simple question in her head (not, how can I always do this right thing myself, but) how can I provide for this right thing to be always done?"
—Florence Nightingale

HOW TO IDENTIFY WHAT NOT TO HAND OFF

Chances are good that much of the information that you were given at the time you began your position is irrelevant (and possibly unhelpful) today. The following comments from the nurse leaders we interviewed suggest that if you focus first on the unchanging essentials and leave your successor with a feeling of hope, you will be setting the new leader up for success:

> "I tried not to pass on negative history, things that can't change. It's water under the bridge."—Deb K.

> "If the structure and foundation was strong, I didn't worry as others already knew and had the information."—Susan B.

> "[I did not focus on] my way of organizing and doing things, as I knew others would create their own way."—Alice S.

"No man ever steps in the same river twice, for it's not the same river and he's not the same man."

—Heraclitus

HOW TO QUANTIFY KNOWLEDGE FOR A HANDOFF

The regulatory nature of healthcare demands that information be transferred correctly and efficiently from one shift to another, from one nurse to another, and from one organization to another. Standard operating procedures, policies and procedures, clinical protocols, and so on create the mechanism for transfer of explicit knowledge. Deb K. states, "In handing off my responsibilities at Children's Hospital, I could easily teach processes—how to budget, names of the people you need to know, who to go to for which type of problem." The deeper difficulty lies in transfer of tacit knowledge—the nuances, intuition, political wisdom, and other intangible elements of relationships.

The importance here is to be prepared for your departure at all times. Nurses get this concept as they realize that the information they hand off each shift must be complete and convey critical patient data so that the next nurse and others on the care team will be able to carry on with information and knowledge to provide safe and effective care—shift after shift. For example, the admitting nurse might not care for the same patient twice. New nurse leaders, however, are essentially caring for *all* of the patients in their organization *all* of the time.

One relatively simple way to be prepared for your transition at all times is to consider the use of a "care and feeding" document. This document compartmentalizes fundamental knowledge a successor would need to know about carrying on your work. Although you can store the information in any word processing or spreadsheet program, you should design the documentation to be easily located (for example, stored on an intranet site), regularly updated, and linked to other relevant documents (for example, internal SharePoint/intranet or external websites). In addition, you should include names of people critical to continuation of your (and others') work. Figure 2.2 shows a slice of an adapted version of a care and feeding document that was created by a system surgical improvement program manager.

CARE AND FEEDING DOCUMENT

Updated _____ by _____

Topic	Information	Resource Contacts
Meetings	Recurring meetings (link to agendas/minutes) Scheduling information (link to Microsoft SharePoint site)	Contact person's email, links
System improvement	Emergency department (link to intranet site) Infection prevention (link to intranet site) Nurse practice (link to intranet site)	Contact person's email, links
Analytics	Surgical improvement (link to SharePoint site)	Contact person's email, links
Electronic medical record (EMR) teams	Process mapping (link to intranet site) Op time (link to intranet site)	Contact person's email, links
Core measures	System site (link to SharePoint site) External website links	Contact person's email, links

Value analysis	System site (link to SharePoint site)	Contact person's email, links
Revenue cycle	System site (link to SharePoint site)	Contact person's email, links

Figure 2.2   Sample "Care and Feeding" Document

Given the rapid expansion of transitions and handoffs expected in the coming years, leader maintenance of these types of "essential knowledge repositories" is clear. McMenamin (2014) shared in his blog:

> The health care and social assistance sector is now projected to grow at an annual rate of 2.6 percent, adding 5.0 million jobs and accounting for nearly one-third of the total projected increase in jobs. By 2022 total employment of RNs and APRNs will increase by 574,400 jobs. In fact, with RN retirements also in the mix, the nation will need to have produced 1.13 million new RNs by 2022 to fill those jobs.

An American Organization of Nurse Executives study (AONE, 2013) estimates that 81% of nurse leaders are over the age of 45 and only 19% of nurse leaders are between the ages of 22 and 44. Given this data and the realization that the numbers of people accessing healthcare will increase, the importance of preparing leaders via solid succession planning programs is critical.

Healthcare organizations need to consider how to keep older nurses engaged in the workforce in non-direct patient care areas as mentors, preceptors, coaches, and consultants. SHRM (2014) reported that the advantages of employing older workers compared to other workers included that they had more work experience, including more knowledge/ skills; they were more mature and professional; they had a stronger work ethic; they were able to serve as mentors; and they were more reliable.

This is critical as the expectation is that the workplace will have a skills shortage, and embracing an older worker strategy is critical for organizational success and knowledge management.

Peg F. notes:

> *An older nurse—someone with a lifetime of experience—can ask lots of questions about the process and challenge a younger nurse with questions that help them understand what they're doing and, more importantly, why they are doing it. Pathways are good for quality, but don't teach common sense.*

As knowledge management systems for nursing evolve, it's important to expand beyond IT-related areas such as e-health, the e-portal, computers, smartphones and tablets, cloud-based storage, SharePoint, and so on. A combination of strategies is critical and must combine explicit and tacit sharing of information and knowledge. Hsia, Lin, Wu, and Tsai (2006) created a framework for knowledge management in nursing in which they used the nursing process to illustrate the critical knowledge management activities and technological functions needed to ensure a thoughtful handoff of critical knowledge. They continued to make the case for integration of nursing practices and knowledge management functions, including knowledge creation, codification transfer, and application, in order to have a relevant knowledge management system while demonstrating the cycle in this process.

"What you leave behind is not what is engraved in stone monuments, but what is woven in the lives of others."

—Pericles

For leaders who have been in a job for any extended period of time, work becomes second nature, and others may marvel at the productivity and the ease with which they perform their work. The term *unconsciously competent* is relevant in this situation. According to Adams (2011), unconscious competence occurs when the individual has had so much practice with a skill that it has become second nature and can be performed easily. As a result, the skill can be performed while executing another task. The individual may be able to teach it to others, depending upon how and when it was learned.

For these individuals, sharing knowledge may be difficult, and they go about their work without effort—they just seem to know what to do without thinking about it. As employees enter an organization, they must learn so much explicit and tacit information. They move from unconscious incompetence to conscious incompetence and conscious competence before reaching the place when the skill is second nature. Given the speed of change, attention needs to be placed on how employees transition through each stage. Without an organized process in place, employees struggle, and a workforce with a high percentage of new team members will struggle with productivity until the skill is mastered. Employing seasoned or retired workers can decrease the learning curve.

PERSONAL APPLICATION

The following questions are designed to help you reflect on the knowledge and wisdom you have gained over your career and to facilitate the successful transfer of this knowledge and wisdom to those nurse leaders who, like you, have devoted their life's work to their patients and to the nursing profession.

1. This chapter described three different types of transitions, including planned transitions (such as retirement), transitions or departures (where less-than-ideal transition planning time is available), and unplanned transitions (such as terminations, death, or acute illness).

   - Which types of transitions applied to each of your career transitions? Which transitions were the most challenging (and why)?

   - Do you have a plan in mind for your planned transition in the event of your retirement or your decision to move to another position with another organization?

   - Who is your successor? Have you begun the formal transfer process?

2. It can be challenging to prioritize content areas for knowledge transfer, particularly if a leader has been in an established position for some time and planning time for the transition is limited.

   - If you decided to leave your current position tomorrow, how might you prioritize content areas for knowledge transfer to others?

   - What content areas rise to the top?

   - What tools would you use to determine information that would be most important to pass on?

3. Facilitating the process of letting go and ensuring a smooth transition for yourself and others can be eased by a more thoughtful and proactive approach.

   - Again, if you decided to leave your current position tomorrow, what steps would you take to prepare yourself—and others—to let go?

   - What actions would you take to facilitate a smooth transition?

   - What are you unconsciously competent about, and how will you go about documenting that knowledge in the event of a transition (planned or unplanned)?

4. Employees born in different generations (veterans, baby boomers, Generation X, and millennials) often have different perspectives on work, including preferences for the way in which they best acquire new knowledge.

   - Describe a situation in which you transferred knowledge to employees who were born in different generations.

   - Did you modify your approach based on their generation?

   - What worked well? What didn't work well?

   - What opportunities do you see to modify your managerial or leadership approach to address generational differences? What approach might you adopt?

LOOKING FORWARD

The challenge of transferring valuable knowledge from one healthcare leader to another is significant, and necessity will be the mother of its invention. We need to build systems that take today's realities into account, including the truth that succession planning will occur in a briefer than ideal time period and that younger leaders' thirst for development and coaching will need to inform the process. Technology will allow us to capture much more essential information than ever before, freeing up opportunities to more deeply consider the transfer of tacit relational knowledge in a more meaningful way and laying the groundwork for the success of future leaders. Leaders will adopt the mind-set that sharing information is power and is an expectation of the role. As the workplace continues to transform and technology provides a repository for explicit information, the culture will accept the truth that "soft" skills are of equal value. Organizations will embrace the reality that employees and organizations are different and will plan for departure upon hire. Transitions will be seamless. Departures will not be about age but about shifting what we want to do with our skills and talents. If the focus remains on retirements, knowledge will flow out of each organization without the methodology to capture it from all employees, regardless of their age. Seasoned workers will help ensure effective knowledge and wisdom transfer. "Effective knowledge transfer is not about leaving a legacy: It's about actually passing on critical 'know-how' and 'know-what' to the people doing that job after you. Leaving a legacy is an important value for veteran employees, and we want them to recognize that" (MacMillan, 2008).

That said, this challenge—although in its infancy—holds the promise of possibility.

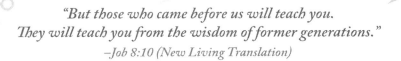

*"But those who came before us will teach you.
They will teach you from the wisdom of former generations."*
—Job 8:10 *(New Living Translation)*

3

ESSENTIAL BUSINESS KNOWLEDGE

JANELLE KRUEGER, MBA, BSN, RN, CCRN
APRIL MYERS, MBA, FACHE

CHAPTER OBJECTIVES

Describe basic business skills that are essential to sustained leadership success.

Provide an example of how unconventional strategic thinking may be key to future healthcare delivery models.

Harness the power of the balanced scorecard as a means to assess goal achievement.

Understand the need for business agreements and contracts.

This chapter is an acknowledgment of the business side to human caring and the basic business competencies all nurse leaders should describe as an expectation of their roles. In the following pages we highlight those tangible business skills that will help all nurse leaders, new or more seasoned, achieve professional goals faster, with fewer setbacks, and increase the value of contribution to the administrative team early on. Some of the skills are technical in nature, some are related to relationships, and still others are related to the importance of continually refining personal attributes.

THE NEED TO SHARE BUSINESS KNOWLEDGE

No longer can nurse leaders rely solely on judgment, traditions, experience, and intuition to justify their decision-making. No longer can nurse leaders completely delegate finance, marketing, and budgeting responsibilities to someone else. Clinical skills alone won't see us through the new paradigm we find ourselves in. The Affordable Care Act (ACA) is accelerating the need for reinvention of care delivery. There is more pressure on nurse leaders and other managers to increase efficiency while improving quality and patient outcomes. There will continue to be many changes in healthcare delivery, and nurse leaders will increasingly be asked to contribute to the strategic planning of new programs. These are skills that can and should be learned, but the business-savvy nurse leaders, who step outside of their comfort zones and learn new ways of working and thinking, will be ready for these challenges and be in the most demand to lead the way.

What follows are examples we have determined to be essential healthcare business knowledge—essential elements that you may not have yet recognized. In some cases, we learned them because of a need to know them, and had we acquired this knowledge earlier in our careers, we would have been a step ahead. In other cases, we discovered this knowledge was part of the core values or habits already entrenched in our DNA, and we now recognize how important those things have been to our success. As you read this chapter, it is important to understand your responsibilities as they exist today and be able to articulate those lessons learned so you can use them as stepping stones in reassuring new leaders as they transition to unfamiliar roles.

LEARNING SPREADSHEET SOFTWARE

Whether you learn Microsoft Excel (or other spreadsheet software) by self-study or through formal classes, you need to learn it. In today's environment, all nurse leaders should expect to incorporate the ability to use spreadsheets effectively into their work requirements. Spreadsheets, which are a mainstay in today's world, both in the workplace and at home, enable you not only to organize data but also to perform financial calculations on that data so you can analyze it and make informed decisions. Financial statements, quality analyses, sortable tables, and performance improvement projects are all dependent on formulas. Get to know how to use the basic functions (predefined formulas) and create formulas, and you will be glad you did. Following are a few critical features and functions, as they are known in Excel:

- Use the Sort command on the Data tab to sort in various ways (ascending, descending, and so on). For example, in a spreadsheet that includes patient names, admission date, the admitting physician's name, and the payer source, the Sort command allows you to quickly sort the contents in a variety of ways: alphabetically by patient name, alphabetically by physician name, chronological by admission date, and so on.

- Create charts and insert trendlines. Displaying data in a well-conceived chart can make your numbers more understandable. Making a chart can often help you spot trends and patterns that may otherwise go unnoticed. A trendline points out the general direction in which the data is going. Sometimes you can forecast future data with trendlines.

- Use the SUM, IF, and ROUND functions to perform common calculations.

- Use the ABS ($) function when you need to use the absolute value of a number. The dollar sign in front of the reference makes it absolute. The $ can be inserted in front of the row or column reference. Generally, when a formula or function is copied and pasted to other cells, the cell references in the formula change to reflect the function's new location (this is called *relative reference*). When the ABS function is used, however, the cell reference does not change when it is copied and pasted to other cells. An example of when ABS is useful is when you need to calculate the same sales tax percentage for products that have different prices. The formula would include $ in front of the cell name with the sales tax. That way that part of the formula never changes.

- Start a new paragraph within a cell by pressing Ctrl+Enter. When writing text in a spreadsheet, this function allows for use of paragraphs within a cell rather than having several sentences blend together.

- The VLOOKUP function searches for a value in the leftmost column of a table and then returns a value in the same row from a column you specify in the table. This function is useful, for example, when creating a position control table where you want to calculate the number of staff needed by skill mix with varying census numbers.

Don't be afraid to use the excuse of wanting to learn more about spreadsheets as an opportunity to connect with other leaders within the organization. Most leaders enjoy a mentoring or coaching moment, and asking for assistance can be an incredible opportunity to build new relationships. As an example, make an appointment with your finance and human resources (HR) colleagues to learn how the position control was developed. This particular topic not only exposes spreadsheet formulas that were used but also makes for easy transition into specific budget questions, such as the following:

- What assumptions were used to create the position control?

- What definition is used for full-time equivalent (FTE)?

- Is the data based on 8- or 12-hour shifts?

- How were the weekday and weekend distributions determined?

- What factor is used to address the nonproductive replacement coverage for each unit?

- How does the position control get updated?

- How does HR use the position control to influence its recruitment efforts?

- How many per-diem/casual staff are incorporated into the position control, and what calculation was used to determine an effective number of per-diem staff?

These questions can easily transition into how the number of nursing hours per patient day (NHPPD) is calculated, how separation of direct and indirect hours is determined, and what assumptions were used for skill mix distribution and RN-to-patient ratios, for example. How does the budget process work and, historically, what has the nurse leader's role been in the process?

Finance people are generally very good with spreadsheets and are often quite willing to teach others. You just have to ask. But do your part by being a good student; practice what you learn and come to the table with pertinent questions that show off the effort you are putting into it. Reviewing your work with a mentor or another colleague helps to better understand your strengths and opportunities but be open to the advice given.

LEARNING TO INTERPRET DATA AND RESULTS

Whether you are reading research articles or looking at the results of a performance improvement project, it's hard to avoid statistics. Every day we encounter people who want us to change the way we do things: update diagnostic equipment, modify employee training programs, add drugs to the formulary, adopt evidence-based practices, sign new contracts with payers, and even reform the healthcare system. People cite statistics from studies to support why we would be better off if we did things their way. Today's decision-makers need to know something about statistics if for no other reason than to deal intelligently with all the studies that suggest changes to something will make a difference in the outcome.

Knowing how to interpret research studies requires some basic statistical skills. Although the quality department is the go-to place for statistical analysis and sophisticated data interpretation, having some basic statistical skills will pay off 10-fold. Consider, for example, when your input helps avoid using a product that ends up having little value or contracting with a vendor who overadvertised the product's value.

Here's another example of why simple data interpretation is critical. Good charts (or graphs) are extremely powerful tools for displaying large quantities of complex data; they help turn the wealth of general information available today into specific knowledge. But, unfortunately, some charts deceive or mislead the individuals reviewing their results. This inaccurate representation of results may happen because the designer chooses to give readers the impression of better performance of results than is actually the situation. In other cases, the person who prepares the graph may want to be accurate and honest, but may mislead the reader by making a poor choice of the graph form or using poor graph construction.

The following items are important to consider when looking at a graph:

- Title

- Axis labels on line or bar charts and section labels on pie charts

- Source of the data and time period

- Uniform size of a symbol in a pictograph

- Scale: Does it start with zero? If not, is there a break shown?

- Scale: Are the numbers equally spaced?

Changing the scale of the graph can alter it. For example, the data in the two graphs shown in Figure 3.1 are identical, but scaling of the Y-axis changes the impression of the magnitude of differences. If a product vendor asked you to order new bed surfaces because of the research results shown in these graphs, what would you do? Quickly comply or challenge the vendor on the marketing ploy? Your patients rely on you to make good choices!

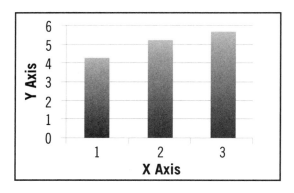

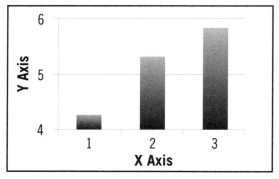

Figure 3.1   Example of Impact of Scale Used in Graphs

CAUSATION VERSUS ASSOCIATION

One of the most important issues in interpreting research findings is understanding how outcomes relate to the intervention that is being evaluated. This understanding involves making the distinction between association and causation and the role that can be played by confounding factors in skewing the evidence.

An *association* exists when one event is more likely to occur because another event has taken place. However, although the two events may be associated, one does not necessarily cause the other; the second event can still occur independently of the first. For example, medical errors may occur by a fatigued nurse. However, even though fatigue may contribute to medical errors, there is no evidence that fatigue directly causes the errors.

A causal relationship exists when one event (cause) is necessary for a second event (effect) to occur. The order in which the two occur is also critical. For example, for scurvy to occur, there must be a deficiency of vitamin C.

Determining cause and effect is an important function of evaluation, but it is also a major challenge. Being able to correctly attribute causation is critical, particularly when conducting an evaluation and interpreting the findings.

IMPROVING YOUR KNOWLEDGE OF TECHNOLOGY

Understanding the use of information technology (IT) to improve the efficiency, safety, and quality of healthcare delivery has become a core competence of nurse leaders. It's hard to pick up a nursing journal these days and not find an article on the rapidly advancing knowledge and technologies in the healthcare sector. Nurses are in a key position of the digital development, regardless of managerial level. Only nurse leaders can ensure that systems meet nursing requirements and needs, not only the formal requirements for documentation but also the professional needs for systems that support the various clinical disciplines as they make real-time patient-care decisions.

Because nurse leaders, at the strategic level, influence the overall decisions in the technology development, it is necessary that nurses with strong nursing, managerial, and informatics skills participate in the entire decision-making process. For nurse leaders to make high-quality decisions, they must collaborate with other clinical disciplines to ensure synergy exists between the various fields of knowledge. That collaboration begins first with having an overall understanding of how technology works in your organization.

Time spent learning how technology works is time well served for nurse leaders who are new to an organization (or new to the role); you should meet with the IT colleagues who can explain the various systems that are used and how they are (or are not) integrated. After getting the big picture from your IT colleagues, set time aside to meet with those care-givers who are considered the "go-to" resources in their area of expertise. They will be the ones to give you the real story on what works well and what needs to get better.

ELECTRONIC MEDICAL RECORDS

In particular, nurse leaders must have a thorough and comprehensive understanding of the electronic medical record (EMR). In fact, in order for nurse leaders to work as advocates for change, they must be able to use and understand the EMR as well as the bedside clinicians with whom they work. Any changes in documentation of care can have a significant impact on nursing practice as well as other clinical depart-ments within the organization. Having a clear vision of why a pathway in the EMR doesn't support compliance to a regulation, why certain data elements must be available to support staff in order to promote pa-tient safety, and why the terminology must support the lexicon used by clinicians makes it paramount that nurse leaders take responsibility for using and understanding the EMR. Simply relying on only those who provide direct care day in and day out to be proficient in the use of the EMR is shortsighted and limits your ability to advocate for your staff and patients.

"May we hope that when we are all dead and gone, leaders will arise who have been personally experienced in the hard, practical work, the difficulties and the joys of organizing nursing reforms, and who will lead far beyond anything we have done."

—Florence Nightingale

EFFECTIVE EMAILS

Another aspect of the technical world that is worth mentioning is email etiquette. There are a number of websites that do a good job of outlining the pitfalls to avoid with email, so we do not cover them all here. There are, however, a few that are important enough to point out; we have learned the hard way that these things can distort the image others have of you and potentially diminish their respect. Often perception is reality; don't let email faux pas be how others define you.

- Stick with the rule of thumb that says, "If you wouldn't say it to someone's face, don't type it in an email." Doing so only makes you look like an uneducated, inconsiderate e-bully.

- Think twice before clicking Reply All. No one wants to read emails from dozens of people when the topic has nothing to do with them. They could just ignore the emails, but many people get notifications of new messages on their smartphones or distracting pop-up messages on their computer screens. Refrain from hitting Reply All unless you really think everyone on the list needs to receive the email.

- Do not write emails in capitals, or all caps. Capitals in emails come across as AGGRESSIVE. Usually this is not the intention of the sender, but nevertheless the recipient can be intimidated by use of capitalization.

In addition to the preceding guidelines, succinct writing is essential to all aspects of communications—whether you're shooting an email to your boss or drafting a formal speech. The goal of writing concisely is to use words that communicate your message as efficiently as possible, a difficult feat for even experienced writers. A technique you can use to guide your communication is the "know, feel, and do" approach. It is one of several similar approaches that came out of education programs "designed to improve communication between patients and health care providers" (National Patient Safety Foundation [NPSF], 2015). The intent was to "encourage patients to become active members of their health care team, and promote improved health outcomes" (2015). Even though the approach was originally developed for verbal communication with patients, the philosophy behind it works with any communication. Essentially it provides an efficient way to have impact on people's behaviors. The following list breaks down the three components:

- *Know—What is the one thing you want the reader to know?*

    Don't get into re-creating the context and trying to explain the big picture. The most important information to get across is how your reader's actions or thinking will change as a direct result of whatever you have to say. Clearly state the one thing that's new and different from the reader's perspective. For example: "Customer satisfaction has dropped, especially in the section *Your Care from Nurses.*"

- *Feel—Why is it important?*

    You can't mandate how people should feel, but you do have to consider the emotional impact you want and determine how to accomplish that. Focus the email content on how you want recipients to see why they should continue to read on—that the content will impact their work. Sticking with the preceding example, "This is important to us on this nursing unit because it is our core business. Our patients tell us that we do not listen to them, we do not explain things in ways they can understand, and we are not treating them with courtesy and respect."

- *Do—What do you want me to do as a result of your communication?*

  Even empowered teammates often need next steps defined fairly explicitly. Without micromanaging their to-do list, detail the suggested and immediate next steps. Most everyone needs help in getting started. Continuing with the customer service example, "We will discuss the results and your feedback in huddles each shift this week. We will take the learnings from those discussions and create a 60-day improvement plan. What we can do immediately is ensure our handoffs include a meet-and-greet with patients and include open-ended questions with patients to get an indication of what they know about their condition and their plan of care."

In summary, it's important to remain professional in company communications, both to appear competent to your customers and because you never know who may intercept your mail. Second, emails that are to the point and easy to read are more efficient. Lastly, employees that understand email etiquette are less likely to put the company at risk (Giang, 2013). Reviewing some of your email communications with a mentor or colleague can be a great way to get feedback on their effectiveness. That objective third party can quickly identify whether you are on track with an efficient, effective message or whether there are opportunities to condense and pinpoint specific messages.

WRITING EFFECTIVE EMAILS

"Joe" is the Lead Infection Control Preventionist for a healthcare organization that has 12 hospitals and multiple post-acute levels of care facilities. He has been working with key stakeholders for a year to purchase and develop an infection control software program that will help automate and streamline across the continuum the process of tracking patient infections. The work has involved analyzing not only infection prevention process workflow but also pharmacy and laboratory departments. There are many departments and people potentially affected by the use of this new electronic tool. For months Joe has been involved in weekly meetings to establish the business requirements for the software as well as identify the measures of success that will be used. Although Joe has reached out to his constituents throughout the process for feedback and input, not everyone with infection prevention responsibilities has been involved. Joe realizes it is now time to send a mass email that will announce the plans for the implementation of the new software.

Using the know–feel–do communication methodology, Joe drafts the following email. Do you agree with its content? Would you recommend he add or eliminate anything?

Great news! St. ABC has purchased Infection Prevention and Control Software to help automate the tracking of infections. Information Systems department representatives and other key stakeholders are in the process of refining the software to support the specific business needs of St. ABC. A workgroup has been created to assist with decisions on design and implementation.

Having the electronic software will streamline the process of tracking, preventing, and managing patient infections and improve quality and safety of patient care. The tool will automate mandatory reporting requirements and enhance the ability for early recognition of potential outbreaks.

Beta sites are currently being identified that will help with testing; otherwise there is nothing you need to do at this time. You will get intermittent emails from me updating you on our progress and ongoing plans.

I hope you are as excited as I am about having access to a tool that will help automate so much of your current paper process.

Joe

HARNESSING THE POWER OF BALANCED SCORECARDS

Healthcare organizations have seen an increase in the utilization of balanced scorecards to detail key strategic goals and metrics. According to a study by Bain and Company (Balanced Scorecard Institute, n.d.), balanced scorecards are among the top 10 most widely used management tools around the world. *Balanced scorecards* are a management system for strategic planning used to align business activities with the overall vision of the organization. The term *balanced scorecard* was coined in the 1990s and can be traced to the pioneering work of General Electric on performance measurement reporting in the 1950s. Balanced scorecard methodology tends to include different business aspects in the document while balancing the key areas such as finance, service, and people (Balanced Scorecard Institute, n.d.). Many organizations believe the philosophy that a greater focus on clinical, quality, and satisfaction will yield greater financial returns. Other organizations believe that the majority of focus needs to be within the finance areas and that other areas may suffer with this philosophy. There needs to be a balanced approach because all the areas are interrelated.

> *"So often people are working hard at the wrong thing. Working on the right thing is probably more important than working hard."*
>
> —Caterina Fake, Flickr co-founder

COMPONENTS OF THE BALANCED SCORECARD

Areas highlighted on scorecards often include financial goals, customer satisfaction metrics, quality measures, growth goals, efficiency metrics, and employee engagement metrics. The following sections review each of these areas as they relate to a hospital balanced scorecard.

Financial Goals

The financial section monitors profitability, revenue growth, and shareholder value by measuring such areas as EBITDARM (earnings before interest expense, taxes, depreciation, amortization, rent, and management fees), total net revenue, cost per patient day, high cost center expenses per patient day, net income, and accounts receivable days.

Customer Satisfaction Metrics

Customer satisfaction focus areas often include results from the HCAHPS (Hospital Consumer Assessment of Healthcare Providers and Systems) patient satisfaction survey. "The intent of the HCAHPS initiative was to provide a standardized survey instrument and data collection methodology for measuring patients' perspectives on hospital care" (Centers for Medicare & Medicaid Services, 2015). The survey was endorsed by the National Quality Forum and given final approval for the national implementation of HCAHPS for public reporting purposes in 2005. There are financial incentives for hospitals to participate in this standardized process that focuses on improved patient experiences. These organizational-specific results are a great tool to gain a better understanding of the customer's perception of the organization. Areas that may be scoring lower than national averages will likely be focus areas or areas that new leaders will need to develop action plans for improvement.

Quality Measures

Hospitals often include their quality metrics within this section as evidenced by national reporting of quality events, such as central line–associated bloodstream infections, hospital-acquired pressure wounds, readmission rates within 30 days of discharge, surgical site infections, and catheter-associated urinary tract infections. There are mandated national quality reporting metrics, and often each state has its own mandated reporting items from a clinical/quality aspect. New nurse leaders need to know how to easily access these state, federal, and regulatory agency reporting requirements to develop their own knowledge base. This awareness and knowledge can certainly minimize risk to their organization.

Growth Goals and Efficiency Metrics

Growth and efficiency are often combined in one section of the scorecard because one factor often drives success or challenges within the other area. A low volume in a service line usually negatively impacts the efficiency and vice versa. Greater volume can help to improve efficiency because fixed costs can be spread out on a higher number. Expenses are often reported as cost per patient day because this calculation can more easily be utilized to compare to budgeted numbers. In scorecards, labor costs are frequently a metric used because labor is almost always the most expensive expense line item for hospitals.

Seasoned nurse leaders often struggle to help new nurse leaders understand the intricacies of staffing models and plans because there are various tools that nurse leaders utilize to manage their labor pool. They may have daily staffing sheets, a master staffing schedule, unit daily staffing assignments, and a patient acuity classification system. Whereas some organizations have adopted an automated staffing tool, most hospitals still schedule their staff using paper tools or spreadsheets. Seasoned nurse leaders can look at a nursing schedule and anticipate potential issues, so a great mentoring opportunity exists for taking the time to ensure new nurse leaders have a thorough understanding of the process. Scheduling the right staff with the right skill mix and competency at the right time is a critical nursing leadership competency. Although most expect scheduling to be a critical competency, many may not anticipate a new leader's potential struggle with developing this skill set.

Purchased services are often a significant expense line item within hospital expenses that can be sucessfully managed. The finance leader can be a great person from whom you can gain an understanding of what services are provided within the organization or which ones are provided by an outside vendor through a contractual arrangement. Leaders need to understand the outsourced vendors, contractual requirements, and expected service standards. Even though the service may be a contracted service, the hospital or healthcare organization still assumes ultimate responsibility for patient care.

Employee Engagement Metrics

Employee engagement is usually a metric on the balanced scorecards because people can be considered the organization's greatest resource. Employee engagement metrics can include such items as employee turnover, key leadership position turnover, employee safety days, and results from employee engagement surveys. Local-level balanced scorecard metric goals often roll up to division scorecard metric goals.

THE BALANCED SCORECORD AS A TOOL FOR SUCCESS

Synergy among departments and employees fosters an overall commitment to the organization's goals. These tools can transform an organization's strategic plan into "marching orders" for the organization on a daily basis. Executives can focus on execution of their strategies and provide governing boards with a one-page scorecard summary. Governing boards can quickly assess the organization's success at a given point in time and make comparisons to other similar business lines within the company.

Most scorecards can be reported on a monthly, quarterly, or yearly time frame. Figure 3.2 is an example of a balanced scorecard. Many scorecards include color-coding to make at-a-glance review very easy. Boxes shown in green typically reference positively meeting or exceeding the metric goal, yellow boxes usually reference results slightly below the goal, and red boxes frequently reflect a signficant negative variance to the goal.

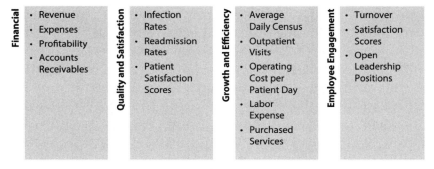

Figure 3.2   Sample Balanced Scorecard

The editors of *Harvard Business Review* selected the balanced scorecard as one of the most influential business ideas of the past 75 years (Balanced Scorecard Institute, n.d.), making it imperative that leaders are comfortable with the tool. Leaders who have this competency can confidently share the organizational goals with their employees while also communicating their potential contributions and expectations. A hospital CEO we interviewed about the balanced scorecard tool in their organization shared the following example about one of their new nurse managers:

> *The nurse manager had thanked the CEO for taking time during one of the leadership meetings to review the year-to-date balanced scorecard. She shared that the scorecard concept had been reviewed in a recent course that she had*

*taken in school, so it was helpful to see her own organiza-
tion's scorecard.*

*The CEO was happy to hear that feedback until the nurse
manager went on to comment that she understood her
area of focus was strictly on the quality area. The CEO
was surprised with that remark and asked for more information on why she felt that way. The nurse manager
shared that she believed that neither she nor her departments were able to impact many of the other areas of the
scorecard. The CEO took time to review each area on the
scorecard to help her know that her day-to-day activities
truly impacted each metric, either directly or indirectly.*

*This exercise was a great learning opportunity for all
parties involved because it gave the CEO the feedback
needed to help connect the dots for all leaders to truly
understand, own, and feel empowered to affect all of the
metrics. The nurse manager felt empowered knowing that
the CEO would take the time to help explain individuals' contributions to the overall organizational success.
This situation was a win-win for all parties involved.*

Taking time to mentor and coach is important so that people can learn
and truly understand; it's a great example of how we can nourish our
young leaders each and every day as they nourish our seasoned leaders
too. Young leaders can help seasoned leaders to be better coaches.

"You can't connect the dots looking forward; you can only connect them looking backwards. So you have to trust that the dots will somehow connect in your future. You have to trust in something—your gut, destiny, life, karma, whatever. This approach has never let me down, and it has made all the difference in my life."

—Steve Jobs

EARLY WINS IN A NEW JOB

Jane Bale, MSN, RN, had just started in her new position of chief clinical officer. She had been successful in her prior role at a different organization, but now she was taking on expanded responsibilities directing multiple clinical departments. She knew making a successful transition was about more than avoiding failure. She wanted to use every opportunity she could to build credibility, demonstrate effectiveness, and leverage her strategic goals. She also recognized her continued success would not only come from early wins but also be a direct result of the quality of the relationships she builds with her key people and the extent to which they would get on board with her new direction. Jane began to reflect on how she might approach this.

Take a moment now to consider the following:

- What kind of questions should Jane think about asking as she meets with various key influencers within the organization?
- Why is it important for Jane to display some vulnerability as she meets with her new team? What can she do that will show her team how much she cares?
- Discuss why understanding her team members' learning styles can help accelerate adoption of her strategic plans.
- What organizational documents might Jane review to get a better sense of the organization's key metrics and performance strategies?

CREATING BUSINESS AGREEMENTS AND CONTRACTS

Up until now we have shared advice meant more for those nurse leaders newly entering into a leadership role or who are finding themselves in a different organization. In those circumstances there is generally a whole organization of people who can be used for learning, obtaining advice, and improving one's efforts. But there is also a whole host of opportunities for experienced nurse leaders who for the first time are considering venturing out on their own and doing independent contractor work. All of the learnings we have reviewed thus far still apply, but the single most important additional advice we can give that pertains to contractor work is to do your homework on the essential elements of a business agreement or contract. Don't be afraid to ask a lawyer to review an agreement you've drafted yourself. If there's a tricky issue you don't feel comfortable handling yourself or an idea you're not sure about, a good small business lawyer can give you drafting advice and get your agreement back on track.

Entering into a business relationship with another party is a serious task with important ramifications and should only be entered into after giving real thought about the relationship you want. Don't fall into the trap of entering into agreements haphazardly or with complete trust of the other party. Even if it's a family member (some would argue especially if it's a family member), the business contract should protect your own business interests first. With that goal in mind, you need to familiarize yourself with some guidelines on how to write a business contract.

According to FindLaw (2013), there are two things to keep in mind when entering or writing a business agreement:

First, does the agreement address all of the possible situations that may arise (or at the very least, the most probable ones)? And second, do the provisions leave too much room for ambiguity? You want the contract to cover the important points and do so in a way that is clear and doesn't leave too much room for interpretation.

The agreement/contract should be accompanied by a cover letter that summarizes the background, expected work, deliverables, timeline, and fees. Use a consulting agreement letter such as the example in Figure 3.3 to provide a succinct overview of the essential elements that the business with which you are entering a relationship can easily interpret.

You can use the following sample letter simply as a guide to identify those key terms and conditions of the transaction. These kind of documents can quickly identify problems (or deal breakers) in the early stages of the negotiations, before incurring the costs of negotiating and performing due diligence work. Being well-prepared can reduce or even eliminate future misunderstandings during negotiations of the defined work. Always seek specialist advice about your specific circumstances so you aren't caught off guard. Being your own boss can be one of the most rewarding ways to share your knowledge and expertise with many others. Start this new adventure by first exploring how others have succeeded. Ask your mentors and colleagues to share their learnings and get their advice.

Company Name
Street Address
City, State, Postal Code

Date

Contact Name
Healthcare Organization
Street Address
City, State, Postal Code

Dear [insert contact name]:

Thank you for the opportunity to provide a proposal to you and your team to strengthen the infrastructure for the nursing team as fully contributing members to the healthcare team at [insert name of healthcare organization]. This work is critical as the challenges of healthcare reform, control of resources, and the full utilization of the scope of nursing continue to dominate healthcare agendas and priorities. The purpose of this letter is to provide a proposal for consultative work with your team over the next 12–18 months. An overview of the work, deliverables, and timelines for this work is included.

As background to the discussions, it was helpful to learn current [insert name of healthcare organization] information. Specifically, [insert name of healthcare organization] includes 20 hospitals in seven states with approximately 20,000 RNs. There are eight hospitals in California. The electronic medical record, [insert name of EMR], was implemented in 2011. The implementation of the EMR illuminated many issues and opportunities for increased consistency and standardization of many processes across the system and clarified the role of nursing in supporting an effective continuum of care for [insert name of healthcare organization] patients. The system is on the Magnet journey. There are eight union contracts within the system. Most recently, [insert name of healthcare organization] was purchased by [insert name of acquiring business], and the system is now in the process of incorporating and merging these two entities.

The goal of the consultation work includes assisting designated leaders at [insert name of healthcare organization] to

1. Create a plan to clarify the role of nursing in the [insert name of healthcare organization].

2. Design an infrastructure and accountability system for interdisciplinary, relationship-based patient care and for selected standardization of care processes.

3. Increase multidisciplinary collaboration, communication, and overall performance across all ministries.

This work will occur over the course of four 2-day sessions (detailed on the following page) occurring each quarter during the next 12 months.

The fees for these services include

- Consultation fee of $ [insert amount] per day
- Travel costs: airfare, lodging, meals, and local transportation (invoiced at cost)

Please contact me immediately with any questions.

Sincerely,

Your Name, Credentials

Consultation Proposal

Phase I (2 days)

Convene Regional CNOs/CMOs to identify goals, assumptions about the changes, and expected outcomes, including:

- Revise the nursing vision to embrace and integrate with the needs of the patient and healthcare system.

- Develop and integrate principles and practices for interdisciplinary, continuum-based patient care, including the patient care delivery model.

- Increase branding clarity for [insert name of healthcare organization] and [insert name of healthcare organization] nursing.

- Select metrics to reflect these goals, including the target levels of performance specific to the continuum of care, patients, staff, and organization:
    - Include both qualitative and quantitative evaluation criteria that measure the relational and business outcomes. Traditional financial metrics to be combined with stories of healing, relationship-based healthcare.

- Co-create (consultant and [insert name of healthcare organization]) a process to develop a team that will assume accountability for dissemination and sustainability of this work.

- Integrate with [insert name of healthcare organization]'s Health Plan/continuum of services.

- Complete a gap analysis specific to goals and current status.

Phase II (1–2 days)

On the basis of Phase I, meet with ENF (Executive Nursing Forum) to evaluate the Phase I information and create a detailed plan addressing individual ministry needs, standardization expectations, and anticipated obstacles/resistors to the plan. Review and affirm selected qualitative and quantitative evaluation criteria that measure both the relational and business outcomes. Traditional financial metrics will be combined with stories of healing, relationship-based healthcare.

This will occur during a 1- or 2-day retreat. ENF members will review the plan with each organization for input, strategies, resistance, and expected outcomes. Each ministry will complete a gap analysis specific to goals and current status.

Phase III (2 days)

Reconvene to discuss feedback from ENF team and review gap analysis between current and desired states, including:

- Develop an implementation and monitoring plan.
- Prioritize work to be done.
- Develop a course-correction plan when obstacles are identified.
- Affirm qualitative and quantitative evaluation criteria that measure both the relational and business outcomes. Traditional financial metrics to be combined with stories of healing, relationship-based healthcare.
- Optimize the use of internal project management resources.

Phase IV (2 days)

Review and analysis of progress and achievement of target goals, including:

- Assure sustainability of the work.
- Discuss needed course corrections.
- Revise gap analysis.

Figure 3.3 Sample Letter for Consulting Agreement

PERSONAL APPLICATION

The following questions are designed to help you reflect on the knowledge and wisdom you have gained over your career and to facilitate the successful transfer of this knowledge and wisdom to those nurse leaders who, like you, have devoted their life's work to their patients and to the nursing profession.

1. Nurse leaders must learn the language of finance in order to maximize collaboration with their finance partners.

   • What spreadsheet software functions do you find yourself frequently using and which ones have you identified that you need to learn?

   • Who was your finance mentor who helped you understand the business aspect of the nurse leader role? What was the greatest learning experience, and how can you share that with those around you?

2. Most organizations use a balanced scorecard approach to assessing goal achievement.

   • How does your organization share the results of its balanced scorecard, or how can you present the idea of such a tool?

   • How do you explain to your staff the importance of the metrics on the balanced scorecard? What do you do to incorporate it into your unit/department operations?

   • As a nurse leader, how might you incorporate your organization's balanced scorecard into your nursing strategic plan?

3. Certain aspects of your nurse leader role involve data analysis and interpretation.

   • Describe an experience when you were caught off guard by the way a chart or graph represented data.

   • How did that experience help you become a better critic thereafter? Why was that important to you?

- How do you use your data interpretation expertise to help others when looking at research articles and deciding if the results are worthy of adopting into your local operations?

4. Email has become a predominant method of communication in today's world.

  - What approach do you use to help ensure your email communication is succinct and effective?

  - Describe an experience at work when someone violated email etiquette and you witnessed the outcome. How did that experience help you become more aware of the power of email and the pitfalls to avoid?

  - Have you ever provided feedback to someone on how the person might have reworded an email to more effectively get the message across? What advice did you give, and how was it received?

LOOKING FORWARD

The need for basic business skills and recognition of the advantages of unconventional strategic thinking should be seen as important stepping stones in the transition of responsibilities to new nurse leaders. As nursing continues to evolve with new hospital structures, fancier gadgets, and political challenges, we must remember the heart of the profession stays the same. Whatever the tools and technologies, the job of the nurse will remain caregiver and advocate for the most sick and vulnerable members of our communities. That is our job one. Never forget it.

> *"There are four ways, and only four ways, in which we have contact with the world. We are evaluated and classified by these four contacts: what we do, how we look, what we say, and how we say it."*
>
> *—Dale Carnegie*

4

ESSENTIAL BUSINESS RELATIONSHIPS

JANELLE KRUEGER, MBA, BSN, RN, CCRN
APRIL MYERS, MBA, FACHE

CHAPTER OBJECTIVES

Describe how learning styles influence ability to process information.

Explain the importance of collaborative relationships among healthcare leaders in the context of succession planning.

Examine the beliefs of a nursing legend specific to nursing value.

For most nurse leaders, understanding the tangible work of the profession is straightforward. Managing pain and monitoring vital signs might be seen as core nursing competencies in most organizations. What is not so clear are the intangible relational competencies necessary to interact effectively with individuals from different cultures, different healthcare professions, and different experiences while still all being expected to achieve the same desired outcomes, namely improved patient health. Every day nurse leaders review staffing levels to ensure patients have the right caregiver at the right time. When patient acuity commands greater nursing time, it is the nurse leader who must justify the need. Finance leaders look to nurse leaders to comply with budgeting expectations. When staffing changes conflict with what was budgeted, the ensuing conversations between the two roles can become one of friction or one of mutual understanding, depending upon the level of partnership and collaboration previously established.

In this chapter, we share wisdom specific to the relational aspects of healthcare, which includes understanding the learning styles of colleagues, knowing where to turn for specific sources of business information about your organization, setting lifelong reading expectations, developing relationships with members of your organization's finance staff, and recognizing and building trust as the glue for sustaining relationships. This chapter concludes with thoughts that Dr. Timothy Porter-O'Grady shared with us about nursing values.

The overriding theme in this chapter is how we can't define the future alone. We need all roles at the table. This means we need mutual understanding and respect to create partnerships with common core values and goals. Only then can we take on the future in such a way that it can be seen as something to look forward to and embrace rather than fear and dread.

UNDERSTANDING LEARNING STYLES

Exceptional leaders are those who strive to be lifelong learners—they have a thirst for new information and challenge themselves making that information applicable in their day-to-day world. Leaders need to have an understanding of how they process new information and how others around them process information. This understanding of learning styles will impact how other leaders will approach them for information and how they may present the information to other nurse leaders. We have heard the phrase "see one, do one, teach one"—lifelong learners are often lifelong teachers and mentors.

A strong understanding of how we accept and recall information offers insight to our learning style. The three learning styles are auditory, visual, and tactile. Auditory learners tend to learn best by listening to lectures, speeches, and discussions. They prefer to hear an explanation of a situation rather than see a diagram or read material. Visual learners tend to learn through sight, which may include presentations, articles, diagrams, or actual demonstrations. Tactile (touch) learners tend to prefer to carry out a physical activity in order to learn new information. This physical activity, through touch, assists them in recalling the new learning.

After you have a basic understanding of these learning styles, you can use what you know about them to identify the learning style of others. Then, by knowing how those individuals you are teaching learn best, you can adapt how you present the information in a format that supports maximum processing and recollection. As an example, consider the situation in which various healthcare professionals would need to learn about (process) a new electronic medical record (EMR) system and then use (recall) that new information. Auditory learners might prefer to listen to prerecorded podcasts, participate in sessions in which people discuss the documentation pathways to use, or listen to lessons learned from other individuals who have recently learned the system. Visual learners might prefer to see recorded webcasts or learning modules that demonstrate the actual pathways and see how the screens advance in the specific documentation pathways. Tactile learners might prefer to learn on the computer, either individually or with others in a computer lab setting, so that they can touch the computer while learning and gaining that understanding.

Meetings provide another opportunity to observe learning styles. Those learners who take copious notes probably lean more toward being visual learners because note-taking enables them to visualize what they are learning. Other visual learners might tend to draw diagrams or create boxes with key words. The auditory learners might not take one note during a meeting, but because they absorb auditory stimuli they might be capturing more information than other people in the same meeting and be able to recall it at a higher rate. Auditory learners tend to prefer environments with limited distractions and background noise, so they are likely to be the people who close a door or window if there are noises coming from the hall or outside. Tactile learners are the people in the meeting who volunteer to work the technology, test a pathway, or control the computer when the group is working off of one spreadsheet.

As you become more familiar with the different learning styles and the habits of the three types of learners, you can quickly get a sense of how your colleagues prefer to learn and gain a greater understanding of other people's learning styles. Although we use all learning styles throughout each situation, people tend to feel most comfortable with one dominant style. Having this understanding increases your productivity, success, and effectiveness in communicating with the various individuals who you come in contact with. For example, if key leaders consistently ask for a copy of the article that you referenced or for the slide deck of a presentation, you might be dealing with a more visual group of learners. If people tend not to take notes and do not ask for any supporting information, they might tend to be more of an auditory group. If the group tends to ask you how to log on to a website you referenced or to come to their office later so that you can show them a computer program, they might have a tendency for tactile learning.

As nurse leaders continue to gain knowledge and prepare to share information, practices, and insight, it is important that they support all learning styles to maximize the learning potential of all of the individuals with whom they interact—colleagues, employees, administrators, and other shareholders, including patients and their families. In addition to improved levels of learning, nurse leaders might notice higher levels of commitment, which can be achieved when people have a strong understanding of new information.

USING BUSINESS DOCUMENTS TO GROW ESSENTIAL BUSINESS KNOWLEDGE

Our learning styles impact how we approach gaining essential business knowledge. Company websites, newsletters, brochures, annual reports, shareholder calls, testimonials, facility tours (either in person or online), and various social media offer insight to an organization. During a review of these sources, you might identify common themes on the organization's key focus areas, such as clinical excellence examples, research programs, employee engagement metrics, and community benefit programs. Even if you will be working at the local level of an organization, it is still important to gain an understanding of the global organization's mission, vision, and values.

After you join an organization or begin working in a consulting role, there are many documents that may be helpful to guide your understanding of the organization. The quality management department may be a great place to ask which key documents the organization uses as guiding documents throughout the year. The quality management department is usually the leader that ensures such key documents are appropriately sent through committees for proper approval, up to and including the governing board. New leaders can also ask their mentors which documents they find themselves referencing frequently.

READ, READ, READ!

Whether it is reading about a couple of mice dealing with the relocation of their cheese (Johnson, 2002), the results of a multiyear Gallup study that explains why organizations go from good to great (Collins, 2001), or the seven habits of highly effective people (Covey, 1989), you need to strive to expose yourself to new ideas and new thinking. Leaders must be readers. Reading and learning from peers within and outside of your industry enable you to grow as an employee, business owner, and leader. Some books will be agonizing to get through. Others will resonate so clearly that you will want to put them on your personal bestseller list. The important thing is that they all stimulate the creative and empathic right brain.

Effective leaders understand the value in continually educating themselves. Whether you reread the same book or article to remind you of concepts or read content on time management and organization as a constant reminder to work on these skills, reading is valuable because it keeps important concepts top of mind. Even reading something you disagree with can have a big impact on your ability to think, both creatively and logically.

Reading can also make you more effective in leading others. Reading increases verbal intelligence, creating more adept and articulate communication. According to Coleman (2012), "Reading novels can improve empathy and understanding of social cues, allowing a leader to better work with and understand others. The resulting heightened emotional intelligence will improve your leadership and management ability" (para. 6).

If you're one of those people who claim you don't have time to read, then make time. Time never "appears" for anything; you have to make it. If nothing else, learn how to multitask around it. Listen to content while driving or walking to work. If you don't have time to read an entire book, read short online articles. If you're dying to read a book but honestly can't find the time, then pair up with a friend and take turns reading and sharing the ideas through short descriptions, or find excerpts of the book online.

If you are a leader, you should strive to develop knowledge to improve yourself, your company, and the people who work for you. To do anything less is to shortchange your ability to lead.

ORGANIZATIONAL CHARTS

An *organizational chart* is a diagram that shows the structure of an organization and the relationships among the various departments and/or roles. Nurse leaders can use this document to get a visual understanding of the organization's reporting structure and as a guide to gain a better understanding of the organization's key leaders. This tool might also aid in identifying potential mentors, business partners, new leaders, seasoned leaders, or even the person who can always solve problems associated with spreadsheet formulas. New nurse leaders can ask their mentors to highlight people on the organizational chart who helped to mentor them and who served as their "go-to" people for various key questions. The tool could help seasoned leaders highlight potential key contacts for new leaders, in addition to those people who easily and readily come to their mind automatically.

The organizational chart also provides insight to the type of organizational structure. Three common models of organizational charts include hierarchical, matrix, and blended structures. Hierarchical models reflect employees reporting to managers who report to other senior managers up to the executives of the organization. Matrix models reflect roles that still show manager level responsibilities but they also integrate regional, national, or global reporting responsibilities through dotted lines to various people. Most organizations have a blended model that supports the overall organizational goals and structure, but the chart still offers insight to the formality of the organization. Hierarchical models tend to present more formal structures with specified chains of command. Matrix and blended models tend to be considered less formal because they support communication throughout various people, departments, and pathways. This is an important piece to understand for succession planning because it could impact how open or encouraged leaders are to mentoring people who may not work directly in their work unit or department. Matrix or blended models may encourage more mentoring across traditional business lines or reporting structures.

Another way to utilize the organizational chart is to share it with new nurse leaders as a way to help them know the leaders within their own clinical areas. They may not have had exposure to such a tool and how to utilize one.

STRATEGIC PLANS

Strategic plans are a potential document that new leaders can utilize to learn about organizations. *Strategic plans* are documents that focus on specialty areas, such as business or quality, or are written as part of an overall organization plan. Strategic plans tend to be written annually, with expected quarterly updates. These annual plans might highlight successes and opportunities reported from the prior time period, and they often outline plans for areas of op-portunities for the future time period. These plans are often standardized documents that are used in each

"Before you are a leader, success is all about growing yourself. When you become a leader, success is all about growing others."
–Jack Welch

facility and across business lines. This standardization creates uniformity for reporting to executive committees and governing boards.

ESTABLISHING COLLABORATIVE RELATIONSHIPS

Many nurse leaders are still attempting to overcome the barriers that hinder a seamless and collaborative relationship between the departments of nursing and finance. It is no secret that a long-standing gap has existed between these two groups, based primarily upon a fundamental difference in spoken language. The stereotype is that finance representatives tend to focus on metrics and bottom lines, whereas nurses make decisions based upon variables that are seemingly less tangible and more unpredictable. The finance leader expects each cost center to comply with the budgeted plan. The nurse leader realizes a patient who needs an unusual number of expensive supplies or needs an extended infusion of an expensive medication will mean the budget may not be met. Nurse leaders must understand that it is their responsibility to be able to explain why a variance occurred and provide ongoing plans to correct the trend.

We recommend you consciously balance your relationship with the chief finance officer (CFO), beginning by being conscious of how much you have to win versus how much you are willing to allow the CFO to win. Then, consider replacing the win-lose relationship with your finance partner with one that is more collaborative, cultivating it in a way that both parties are equally engaged in planning and problem-solving. Approach this relationship as a partnership in which you have enough confidence to understand when you will allow yourself to be influenced rather than digging in your heels.

Think about working with your financial support person as if there are three phases to data analysis and assessment that keep your department on track with set goals. These phases include the proactive phase, the concurrent phase, and the retrospective phase, which are described in the following sections.

THE PROACTIVE PHASE

In the proactive phase, you need to think about what you want your department to achieve in 3 or 4 years. As part of the process of identifying these departmental goals, you should consider what you need financially to get there: What kind of capital expenditures will be needed? Will you require a change to the delivery model or skill mix used? In addition, you need to link the desired goals to trended data and outcomes as much as possible. For example, if it has been determined that your transitional hospital will start taking and caring for transplant patients, and one of the goals set for this patient population is to keep the patients from returning to the short-term acute care hospital because of a change in condition, it would be imperative for you to present a plan for how nurses will be trained and deemed competent to care for and manage this new patient population. That means extra nonproductive hours needed for education and training, perhaps more registered nurses on the position control because of the increased ratio needed for this high-acuity patient population, and more monitoring equipment (capital expenditure). Understanding these needs and having a detailed execution plan help make for a smoother transition and building a budget that allows for this change.

Whenever possible, get involved in forecasting the budget at the very beginning. Planning forces you to look at future services and the direction healthcare is moving to make educated, evidence-based, sound business decisions. As with your home budget, your work budget must include information that enables you to predict incoming revenue and evaluate your healthcare environment to help you plan where to best allocate those dollars. And if your department gets passed up for some other project, be ready to explain how that could change the outcomes for the department and also for the organization and its patients. The best tactic is one of trying to create the future rather than just living with what happens. Despite the obstacles and setbacks, don't give up on the long-range plan.

Given the amount of clinical and financial data that is now available, a core competence for the nurse leader now includes the ability to read, interpret, and manage the data to guide effective decision-making. Nurse leaders must become comfortable with reading and analyzing spreadsheets, trendlines, and graphs. There is no substitute for information in an age of voluminous data.

THE CONCURRENT PHASE

Management of ongoing activities includes comparing the actual spending to the budgeted amounts and making adjustments accordingly. For example, monthly reports might be generated to compare what was budgeted for staffing and operational supplies in comparison to what was actually spent. Nurse leaders must receive this information in a timely manner so they can justify any variance between the budget and actual amounts and make necessary adjustments.

Further, nurse leaders are accountable for keeping abreast of what's going on and in what direction the data might be shifting. Clearly explain to your finance colleagues what data is important to you as well as why it is important. Don't accept some cookie-cutter report if it isn't helping you make better decisions. Finance leaders are often most aware of the data elements that make up prebuilt queries and reports. If they know what you are looking for, chances are they can work it into a standard report.

THE RETROSPECTIVE PHASE

Even with all the planning that you do, things might still happen that result in overruns, redos, and/or adverse outcomes. When these events occur—and they certainly will—do your best to avoid becoming overly defensive. Instead, state the facts as you understand them and work with your finance partner to discuss the reality of the situation and develop a plan to fix it. If necessary, engage in a conversation about potentially finding funds from other areas so as to continue with a revised plan. Peter Drucker (1996) predicted, "The leader of the future will be a person who knows how to ask" (p. 279). Leaders who ask for input on a regular basis are seen as more effective.

AN UNLIKELY PARTNERSHIP

We all know that delivering quality and safe patient care now takes a village more than it ever has before. And creating that village of care-givers is dependent on building and maintaining many relationships—including relationships with financial partners who are not directly involved in caregiving at the bedside. Sometimes our best relationships with finance partners happen in unusual ways, such as in the story we're about to share, and sometimes dedication to our cause comes from un-likely sources. Take the story of "Bill," for example, who was the CFO where Janelle Krueger (this chapter's co-author) worked:

> Bill was the CFO of the hospital for 10 years. Others saw Bill as the stereotypical finance person—a numbers cruncher locked in his office with the sole purpose of applying policies and procedures and saying "no" to any request that cost money.

But that was about to change for Bill. You see, the hospital embarked on a new approach to leadership rounding. Each department leader—whether clinical or nonclinical—would visit patients and families as a way to obtain valuable feedback, initiate any needed service recovery, and bring a different set of eyes and ears to the patient's bedside on a regular basis.

The news of this approach paralyzed Bill. He had barely ever entered a patient's room before, much less talked to patients and their families. He didn't know what to say, what to look for, or how to begin building relationships with patients. To lessen the fear, each nonclinical leader was paired with a clinical leader, and the pair would round together. I was paired with Bill.

During the first few days of rounding, Bill mostly stood outside patient rooms, watching me interact with the patients. He heard me ask patients simple questions such as, "How is your stay going so far?" "Has your physician been in today?" and "Is your pain being managed?" He observed me looking at the environment to identify potential hazards, checking to see whether the correct date was on the white board and verifying that needed equipment was present and working.

During the second week of rounding, Bill felt comfortable enough to enter the patient rooms with me and actually ask some of the questions himself. If he couldn't answer questions he knew he had me to help respond. As we rounded together, I began to explain to Bill the patient's environment: the purpose of equipment, the importance of having the correct information on the white board, and the insight that could be gained by getting to know the stories of some of the patients.

Four weeks into our new approach to leadership rounding, Bill was actually enjoying some of the conversations he was having with patients and their families. There was one patient in particular that Bill kept his eye on, "Miss Parkerson." Miss Parkerson was one of our sicker patients. She needed a ventilator to breathe, she had a large wound, and she was generally uncomfortable. Every day that we would visit Miss Parkerson, Bill would ask what else I thought we could do to help her be more comfortable. You could tell he was saddened by how little progress she was making and wondering why we couldn't do more. Over the weeks, we learned from Miss Parkerson's family that she had special lotion she used at home to help with her dry skin. She would use that lotion, especially on her feet, because her feet irritated her the most when that skin got dry and brittle.

One day, I got pulled away during our rounding to address some staff questions. When I caught up to Bill, I found him in Miss Parkerson's room. He was at the foot of the bed rubbing her feet while humming a soft tune. He was so focused on what he was doing he didn't even see me arrive. He just kept gently rubbing Miss Parkerson's knotted, worn feet, his eyes closed as he hummed the song. The room felt completely different. There were no alarms ringing, no television blaring, and no patient agitation, just calmness and peacefulness. That was something I hadn't seen in this room in a long time.

When Bill was done, we left the room and I asked him to share his experience. It turns out, the day before, he had met with the wound care nurse to ask her what kind of lotion would be beneficial for Miss Parkerson's feet and still be considered an appropriate part of her plan of care. The wound care nurse had given Bill some options that he wrote down, took to the local drugstore, and purchased on his own. That was what he was using when I saw him in her room that day. No one asked Bill to do it. He just did it on his own out of human kindness and caring conscientiousness.

Some may say that leadership rounding changed Bill. But I believe leadership rounding simply brought out in Bill his real self—a caring self that was never before given the opportunity to be expressed. The purposeful design of leadership rounding to include participants who historically were not involved in patient care was transforming. The village just became bigger...and better. The village now had more people to listen, more people to observe, and more people to intervene.

Not only did Bill listen, observe, and intervene with patients, but he also began to notice the "business" of running a unit. He heard staff members explain to others that they couldn't comply with personal protective equipment expectations because they had run out of gowns; there just weren't enough ordered to keep supplies at the levels needed. He also saw the frustration on nurses' faces when equipment broke down and replacements weren't readily available.

As Bill learned what it meant when equipment didn't work and when supplies weren't sufficient, he asked to join the patient safety and environment of care meetings so he could get more involved in addressing concerns. He became an advocate for the patients and staff. And I got a new leadership partner in Bill. Our work collaboration only got better and stronger. We appreciated more the strengths each of us brought to the table, and we always made time for each other.

I share with you Bill's story because it is a wonderful example of what can happen when we build relationships with people who might be unlikely allies simply because of titles or positions. Everyone wants to learn and have value. Bill's value grew 10-fold because he took advantage of an opportunity to better understand the core business. Because others were patient and allowed him to progress slowly at his own pace and comfort level, he became a star in the eyes of all staff. If Bill would have been ridiculed at the start of this adventure because of his lack of comfort, he might never have gotten to where he is today. Impatience early in interactions can set the tone for the long-term relationship. There were so many wins gained by not being quick to judge and by executing that age-old leadership theory of "being on all the time." Staff saw how I worked with Bill and could relate it to similar situations they had with a newly hired nurse or a patient's challenging family member. The experience brought a new perspective to the importance of nourishing those around us.

FOSTERING TRUST AND TRUSTWORTHINESS

The business of healthcare has many stakeholders: patients and their families, employees, vendors, physicians, and more. To be effective healthcare leaders, we must build relationships with our stakeholders so outcomes are productive and trust is fostered. Trust is the foundation of all relationships, and that includes leadership and followership. Without trust, no leadership happens in the relationship. Relationships fall apart, and the organizational culture becomes one of every man for himself. Experience and wisdom are lost, organizations fail, and patients suffer.

Stephen Covey (1989) tells us that trust is a function of two things: character and competence. Both are vital to building relationships. A person may seem genuine and sincere, but you won't fully trust that person if he or she doesn't demonstrate ability. Honest people who are incompetent in their area of professed expertise are not trustworthy. Trustworthiness is more than integrity; it conveys competence.

Leaders must spend a lot of time investing in building trust in their followers. Achieving trust is not about mastering techniques to win people over; it's about living a life full of integrity and honor and truly gaining the respect of followers. Learn to trust and learn to be trusted.

BUILDING YOUR CHARACTER

Trust is based on a very simple principle. Will you do what you say? Do your words count for something? If you're a person who cannot seem to live up to what you say, you have to consciously work at it. Before you can expect others to trust you, you have to trust yourself that you will do what you said you would. Learn to develop consistency in word and action. Character is built before relationships.

BEING OPEN TO TRUSTING OTHERS

Before you can expect others to trust you, you as a leader must first be ready to trust others. Trusting others means you don't micromanage their behavior or activities; it means you delegate your authority to them; it means you support them even when their truth is not what you want to hear. All these actions give your followers assurance that you, indeed, trust their ability and character.

RECOGNIZING THAT TRUST TAKES TIME

It takes a long time to build trust and only seconds to destroy it. As you lead, it is in the small events where you display your credibility that results in long-term trust and respect. Arriving on time or keeping a promise that may be hard to fulfill means so much more than what might be evident on the surface. And with that trust you will find that you have an effective team that moves fast and works closely together.

"The key to successful leadership today is influence, not authority."
–Kenneth Blanchard

Nurses spend the greatest amount of time with consumers of healthcare. This situation places them in a position to influence lifestyles. Getting patients to seek further assistance or follow advice may depend on the quality of the nurse–patient relationship. Trust in a work relationship means you believe your colleagues are well-intentioned toward you, that they "have your back." You can rely on them to do what they say they'll do; you believe you'll have their support in managing the demands you face at work. Additionally, trust is just as crucial in developing collaborative relationships between nurses and professionals in other healthcare disciplines to ensure effective team functioning. That level of trust is the foundation upon which financial and quality success can be built. Trust is a key component in a healthy work environment. In healthcare facilities where trusting work relationships exist, more work gets done and it gets done in an effective way. That's where the value proposition comes into play. In other words, value cannot be achieved without collaboration, partnerships, and trust.

INSIGHTS FROM A LEGEND: AN INTERVIEW WITH TIM PORTER-O'GRADY

Increasing the knowledge and clear demonstration of the value of nursing within the marketplace continues to be a challenge for those in the nursing profession. We asked Dr. Timothy Porter-O'Grady to share his thoughts on creating more clarity on the value of nursing. Porter-O'Grady is a seasoned nurse executive who has published extensively. He is recognized worldwide for his work on interdisciplinary shared governance models, clinical leadership, conflict, and health futures. We thought there was no one better to offer insight on what today's nurse leader must think about as the industry defines the value of nursing in this time of the consumer's focus on ensuring quality on dollars spent. Following are some questions posed to Porter-O'Grady and his practical yet thought-provoking responses (T. Porter-O'Grady, personal communication, May 28, 2015).

DEFINING VALUE

Porter-O'Grady reminds us that the notion of value can be very difficult to define and has been a long-term conundrum. He shares that as we move toward a value-driven health delivery system, where value is defined within the context of service excellence, meeting defined quality metrics, and affordability, focus needs to be around the notion of how we participate in that measure of value. Delineating nursing value may be broader than the value equation that may be quantified as a direct impact value to the organization. The whole notion of nursing value could be broken down into the two areas: How do we play out our role, and what is our contribution as a partner in the collective delivery of care?

Porter-O'Grady goes on to say that historically, leaders have focused on individual impact. Contributions can vary significantly depending on the aggregate delivery of care model and how one may define or distribute the dollars associated with that care. In the future, care will be bundled into different categories, such as episodes of care, care for particular populations, or care along the health continuum. The future work for nursing leaders is to define what nurses do as a partner in the overall contribution of value in each of the bundled areas. This approach will serve as the foundation for how we delineate the value of care.

ACCOUNTING FOR THE WORK OF NURSING

Porter-O'Grady shared his opinion on those proposals that include using nursing intensity billing, where nursing would be considered a billable expense rather than a service that is incorporated into room and bed charges. Nursing intensity billing is based on models that might not be as pertinent today as they were in the past. He shared that although there are several articles that reference the need for higher levels of nursing intensity, there has not been success in charging higher prices or commanding higher reimbursement from payers. There has not been the interest by the payers because there has not been demonstrable evidence that outcomes improve with additional staffing. Future consideration should include clarity of the nursing role within the Triple Aim and clarity of the nature of the partnership that is involved in a particular bundle of care. This consideration may determine a calculation of price to be paid for that care. In the future, nurse leaders will need to calculate value in the measure of contribution, percentage of contribution to the whole, and the contribution margin for the price that was agreed upon in relation to the sum of the cost of the parts. This financial algorithm can be a strong approach for looking at pricing and also for quantifying the competency of the staff because there is a direct correlation between staff competency and the capacity to delineate an impact.

Higher numbers of full-time equivalents (FTEs) do not always correlate to higher levels of service or improved outcomes. New nursing leaders will need to continue to broaden their knowledge to approach the value of nursing in a very different way. Seasoned leaders will need to be open to learning new approaches so that new value-driven service delivery models can be considered. All nursing leaders need to be able to articulate the role of nursing within their organizations, both with regard to the present and to what the future might look like. Although the conversations might be very different in each organization, it is the responsibility of all nursing leaders to be prepared to have this value conversation within their organization.

QUANTIFYING VALUE

Porter-O'Grady explained that nurses taking a more active role in learning about quantifying how their work makes a difference in the value-based delivery system is an opportunity to encourage nurse leaders to be involved in their local professional organizations in order to stay aware of current events and to encourage peers to consider new approaches. Many organizations, such as the Institute for Healthcare Improvement (IHI), American Hospital Association (AHA), Medical Group Management Association (MGMA), American Organization of Nurse Executives (AONE), and Healthcare Information and Management Systems Society (HIMSS), have national conferences that now emphasize creating new value models for advancing health. Porter-O'Grady shared that many of these conferences have sessions dedicated to showcasing new delivery models and the impact on their organizations, providers, and patients.

We recommend that you research your organization's tuition reimbursement program or, if you are joining a new organization, you negotiate your attendance at a relevant conference each year. Taking advantage of such opportunities helps to ensure that you are continuing your education.

MEASURING VALUE

Porter-O'Grady shared that metrics will continue to be a key part of measuring value in healthcare. Many nurse leaders trust the processes that are in place and get frustrated when outcomes cannot be achieved. The focus needs to be on reviewing the process to determine if it's relevant and to ensure that the expected outcomes can be achieved. Organizations often increase the metrics that they are collecting if a process is not working. Yet collecting more data will likely not improve the process unless time is spent on truly understanding the process to determine the cause-and-effect relationship in light of its impact on outcomes. Nursing leaders often represent a notion that working harder will create better outcomes. Sometimes the work is labor-intensive but is not having any impact on improvement. The productive solution might actually be to work less but make sure the work done is relevant and demonstrates an impact. Now, this might go against everything that we have learned because we are conditioned to think that we must work harder or longer hours to make a difference. We all know people who might work long hours without having any more impact than others who work fewer hours.

Porter-O'Grady went on to explain that this strategy of working more relevantly can help support the work/life balance that many of us strive for each and every day. At the end of a week, reflect on how you used your time. Questions to ask yourself may include, "Did my work add value to my department or organization?" "Did I proactively schedule my time to ensure priority for important areas?" and "Did others control my calendar because I had not proactively scheduled time for these relevant activities?" These questions should help guide you to planning the following week to ensure that the calendar reflects important and relevant work. If your calendar does not reflect what is important, you will likely be trapped by minutiae and find that you do not accomplish meaningful objectives.

DEVELOPING A REFLECTIVE CAPACITY

Again, Porter-O'Grady reminds us that times are certainly changing, and this can be a very exciting time as leaders across the continuum focus on the Triple Aim by enhancing the patient experience, having a positive impact on the health of the population that we serve, and creating a sustainable price for the care that is provided. Strong leaders need to develop a strong reflective capacity. Porter-O'Grady describes *reflective capacity* as an ability to understand what has worked and what has not worked. Seasoned nurse leaders can use this reflective capacity to mentor new nurses. New generations come with their own strengths, such as a lack of presets and lack of awareness of past constraints. The conversation needs to take place between seasoned nurse leaders and new generations so that they can respect each other's strengths to build the future. Each group needs to make themselves present and available to hear people's stories about their experiences that have brought them to the leader that they are today. Everyone has gifts to share with others, and we may not realize the impact of that gift until later in our careers. We might recall a certain story shared earlier in our career when we find ourselves in a similar situation. In the reflective conversation between the experienced and the new nurse, an emerging and valuable point of reference can be arrived at that provides an opportunity to be mutually supportive and committed to learning and growing together.

UNDERSTANDING THE DIFFERENCE BETWEEN OUTPUT AND VALUE

Porter-O'Grady shared the concept of "ignorance of innovation," which can also be considered a special gift. This lack of experience can serve as an opportunity for the unknown to contribute an insight that has never been shared before. Seasoned leaders bring the gift of the *wisdom of time*, another term Porter-O'Grady uses. When all of these leaders connect, great things can happen as they share their ideas and passion for the work that they do. All levels of leaders can have an impact on creating the future of healthcare, so we challenge you to get involved, question the current processes, and believe that every single person can make a contribution to impact tomorrow.

Porter-O'Grady shared that he believes no one has a greater effect on health than a nurse, so he encourages nurses to do what is right in transforming the healthcare system through intentional work that ultimately advances the health of our society. This intentional work will help ensure a seat at the table for nursing leaders within all organizations. Time is our most precious resource, so use it wisely to help align the relevant work in defining our value and creating a better tomorrow.

PERSONAL APPLICATION

The following questions are designed to help you reflect on the knowledge and wisdom you have gained over your career and to facilitate the successful transfer of this knowledge and wisdom to those nurse leaders who, like you, have devoted their life's work to their patients and to the nursing profession.

1. The three primary learning styles are auditory, visual, and tactile.
   - Which learning style seems to be more effective for you?
   - Identify a situation when you struggled understanding the concept because your learning style wasn't used. What would have changed had your primary learning style been used?
   - How might identifying the primary learning styles of your team members be important early on in a project? Can you accurately identify your team members' learning styles? If not, how can you make this happen?

2. There are a number of business documents that are the foundation to defining what an organization is and what is important to that organization.
   - Name several business documents you look to when newly hired to help you better understand the company's strategy, key metrics, and potential mentors or partners. How can you ensure these are available?
   - As a nurse leader, who is the first person you reach out to in a new organization to help you better understand the culture and expectations?

3. It is said that nurse leaders need to establish a collaborative relationship with their finance partners.
   - What are the key measures for which you want you and your finance partner to have mutual understanding and perspective about?
   - Describe a situation when you and your finance peer were not on the same page. What happened, and could it have been avoided?
   - How often do you find it important to meet with your finance partners and why?

4. Successful teamwork is built on a foundation of trust.

- As a leader, what do you do to invest in building trust in your team members? Do you believe that you currently have it?

- Why is it important in business for relationships to be based on honesty, trust, fairness, and respect?

- Think of a time when you had a boss or team leader who kept key pieces of information to himself or revealed it to only some team members. What did that behavior do to the common understanding of the issue and the ability to create the trust needed for effective and sustainable engagement?

5. "Ignorance of Innovation" can be a special gift.

- Describe a situation where a nurse newbie came forward with a great idea or great insight into an ongoing issue. How did others respond to that nurse and the presented idea? Was this an opportunity for you to handle the situation differently?

- Why is it important that in today's turbulent healthcare world, we need to demand that all nurses, from novices to experts, come forward with innovative thinking and contributions?

LOOKING FORWARD

"If desperation is the mother of innovation, then ignorance might be its father" (Tjan, 2010). This quotation means that great creativity and innovation often come from those persons who have not yet been subject to experience and bias. Using this insight along with Porter-O'Grady's reference to "ignorance of innovation," nurse leaders would be wise to approach the future with an understanding that the novice nurse can be a great contributor to a new and innovative approach to the delivery of patient care. The Affordable Care Act (ACA) is seeking to intertwine quality of care with the cost of care. Reducing cost is not enough. Nurses are fundamental to the success of emerging patient-centered care delivery models that will achieve such desired quality goals. Coordinating and integrating care across settings and providers, embracing prevention and wellness care, promoting patient and family education and involvement in their own outcomes, and advocating chronic disease management are all essentials of nursing practice. In these areas of expertise, nurses can serve as leaders and teachers to our interprofessional colleagues and together can streamline the path of patients through the system, selecting treatment approaches that improve outcomes while eliminating services that do not. The future will be a new way to deliver healthcare as a result of innovative thinking from the novice to the expert.

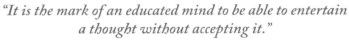

"It is the mark of an educated mind to be able to entertain a thought without accepting it."

–Aristotle

5

THE ART AND SCIENCE OF KNOWLEDGE & WISDOM TRANSFER

JENNIFER MENSIK, PHD, MBA, RN, NEA-BC, FAAN
JENNIFER SCHOMBURG, MHA, MA

CHAPTER OBJECTIVES

Understand how personality plays a role in passing/receiving information.

Describe the four components of the VARK approach.

Understand how being an introvert or extrovert might influence your perception.

Recognize the effect different intelligences might play on passing/receiving information.

Describe the difference among knowledge, wisdom, and insight.

Explore one method for finding common ground.

For those individuals who are part of Generations X and Y, the receiving of knowledge—particularly from members of previous generations—may be anything but an appreciative or inviting experience. The younger generations may feel, for example, that the knowledge being shared is a specific demand or command that must be carried out in a specific manner as opposed to recognizing the knowledge as a collection of valuable information and data gleaned over time and experience from the individuals handing off the knowledge. Individuals from the silent or baby boomer generation might feel as if the younger generations do not appreciate their experience or that the younger generations do not listen even though they are in their own ways. Many times these perceptions are a result of generational differences and, notably, the differences in the various generations' communication styles. All generations need to find common ground and work together to hand off knowledge in a way that facilitates and promotes growth and development for everyone.

An important step in this process is to understand that there is an art and science to handing off and receiving knowledge. Some information and skills can be handed off through a formalized set of principles and guidelines one might find in a set of policies or articles. Other information may be less formalized and often intuitive and ambiguous as the receiver is not sure of the applicability yet (which is what makes it *knowledge* as opposed to *information*, as we will discuss later in this chapter). To further complicate the issue, information for one generation is often used in different ways than it was used in prior generations. Technology is valued and used differently across generations, so it is important to consider these implications for handing off knowledge between younger or older generations. Most of the issues between generations, in our opinion, are due more to lack of understanding personality and communication styles than the year in which the individuals were born.

This chapter provide guidelines for handing off knowledge to different generations, makes suggestions for seeking out and receiving knowledge from older generations, and offers strategies on how to share knowledge through avenues that capitalize on every generation's perspectives.

THE DESIRE FOR KNOWLEDGE TRANSFER

People have a desire to connect. One way to connect to others is through passing knowledge to another person. The urge to pass along knowledge—that which seems important or uniquely gained information—to the next person or generation is strong. People want to leave a legacy: They want to be remembered in some way, and they want to know that their life's work is not in vain.

Prior to tweets, texts, blogs, endless Internet searches, and even books there was simply the spoken word, frequently thought of as storytelling. Learning styles and attention deficit and hyperactivity disorders (ADHD) were not taken into consideration yet. Hours were spent sitting around fires learning about ancestry, moral values and norms, theories on how the world came to exist, and ever-important survival skills. Much information has been lost as its applicability has decreased. How are we to ensure that the pertinent information of our time is passed along to future generations? Who is qualified to determine what is deemed applicable? Part of the answer to these questions is through understanding the art and science of passing on knowledge.

STORYTELLING AS THE ART

Storytelling might be viewed as the art of passing along knowledge. Storytelling can be tracked back through artwork scratched on cave walls, carved into clay tables, and weaved into beautiful textiles. The best storytellers were those who could keep the audience's attention for long periods of time without the audience noticing that they were learning anything or being led through a thought-provoking exercise. We just enjoy listening to stories. The art of storytelling eventually gave way to a more formalized method of educating the masses. Yet the best teachers still seem to be those who are able to entertain large groups of students who have varying levels of interest, intellect, and backgrounds. These teachers appeal to their audience.

Storytellers evaluated the crowd's interest by paying close attention to body language. There were no standardized tests to verify the knowledge gained by the audience. There was simply applause, nods of approval, or deafening silence to signify approval or distaste for the storyteller's craft. Such is art. It is subjective and sometimes lost on those who do not appreciate it for what it is.

SCIENCE OF HANDING OFF KNOWLEDGE

The science of handing off knowledge relies upon the interest of and an action from the exchanging parties. This handing off of knowledge from one generation to another might look much like the passing of the baton between runners in a relay race. The most important part of the race, where the race can be lost or won, lies in the handoff of the baton. Important milliseconds can be gained or lost during this crucial exchange. If this exchange is perfected, the team wins. If there is a misstep, the team loses.

Take a moment to picture in your mind what the handoff of the baton looks like. The runner in front, the receiver of the baton, is actively reaching back, stretching with all of his might to take the baton and carry it to the next runner on the relay team. The runner in back, the giver of the baton, is lunging forward to the extent of his ability to pass along the baton. Both parties actively participate in the passing of the baton. And so it must be with the givers and receivers of knowledge. The givers must be willing to share and stretch beyond their comfort zone to successfully pass along insights. The receivers of knowledge must be willing to reach out and accept the knowledge in the method in which it is given.

LEARNING STYLES AND KNOWLEDGE TRANSFER

Although there might be differences between generations, it is important to note that there are also commonalities, such as learning style, that are universal to individuals; those commonalities are not specific to the generation to which they belong. The term *learning style* is broadly used to indicate how "learners gather, sift through, interpret, organize, come to conclusions about and store information for further use" (Chick, 2015).

The Sensory approach to learning, or the VARK approach, is one of the most well-known learning styles. VARK stands for Visual, Aural, Reading/writing, and Kinesthetic. This approach theorizes that visual learners grasp a concept by seeing it; aural learners by hearing the information; reading learners by, you guessed it, reading the information; and kinesthetic learners by actually performing the task that is being taught (Chick, 2015). Therefore, if you like to tell stories, you need to assess the learning style of the person receiving your knowledge. For example, with learners of the reading type, you can tell your story, but for the best outcome tell it through writing instead of verbal communication.

The Personality approach to learning, or the Myers-Briggs Type Indicator (MBTI) approach, is based on distinct psychological types categorized by C. G. Jung and operationalized by I. B. Myers and K. C. Briggs. The MBTI measures four separate preferences (known as *indices*), each of which is based on Jung's theories concerning perception, processes, and attitudes (O'Brien, Bernold, & Akroyd, 1998). The four indices are judgment/perception, extroversion/introversion, thinking/feeling, and sensing/intuition.

There are 16 possible combinations of learning styles under this model. After determining the individual's style, you know how to tailor your communication for that individual based on his or her set of preferences. Examples include:

- Hold a face-to-face meeting outside the employment setting.

- Send written information in advance so that the individual has the opportunity to think about something on his or her own before having a face-to-face meeting.

- Allow time for small talk; get to know the individual personally.

- Allow the individual time to think; do not expect an answer to a new issue immediately.

- Tailor the ratio of face-to-face to email communication toward the individual's preference, not just the leader's preferred communication style.

- Recognize that the individual may not speak up at a large group meeting and that smaller group meetings may be preferable.

Think about where you fit on this model and where the person you are mentoring fits best. Passing knowledge is not a one-way street, and acknowledging base differences makes the process easier! If you are an extrovert and the person you are passing knowledge to is an introvert, are you taking the person's aloofness as a sign that he or she does not care?

Recognize that the person might need time to think about what you said in order to understand how it fits in his or her own life.

INFORMATION PROCESSING: INTROVERTS VERSUS EXTROVERTS

Extroverts tend to "think" by talking aloud and introverts often "think" without saying a word. Have you ever been in a meeting where the extrovert talks and talks and talks? Throwing out idea after idea, often seeming to change her mind? It drives introverts crazy because it seems like the extroverts are being inconsistent when really they are just "thinking through things"—out loud, of course! And of course, the silent introverts appear aloof—partly because they are working on processing information in their heads. This behavior can drive extroverts crazy because they want introverts to engage in their thinking out loud—the brainstorming.

How do we help each other? Remember this:

- **Introverts.** Give extroverts time to talk or "think" out loud. Whether you are passing information on to them or receiving it, extroverts need to talk about it to process it. Don't judge their talking!

- **Extroverts.** Give introverts time to think silently by themselves. If you are requesting information from them or giving them knowledge, introverts will process it without talking out loud. Don't judge their silence!

Also, keep in mind that shyness is not an introvert trait. Plenty of extroverts are shy in new situations or with new people!

The Aptitude approach to learning, also known as the Theory of Multiple Intelligences, was developed by Howard Gardner, PhD, professor of education at Harvard University. Although Gardner's early work consisted of six intelligences, the theory now consists of nine intelligences—and there is the possibility that others may expand the list. "These intelligences (or competencies) relate to a person's unique aptitude set of capabilities and ways they might prefer to demonstrate intellectual abilities" (Armstrong, n.d., p. 1). See Table 5.1 for the names and descriptions of these intelligences.

TABLE 5.1: THE NINE INTELLIGENCES THAT COMPRISE THE THEORY OF MULTIPLE INTELLIGENCES

Intelligence Type	Description
Verbal-linguistic intelligence "Word smart"	Well-developed verbal skills and sensitivity to the sounds, meanings, and rhythms of words
Logical-mathematical intelligence "Number/reasoning smart"	Ability to think conceptually and abstractly with a capacity to discern logical and numerical patterns
Spatial-visual intelligence "Picture smart"	Capacity to think in images and pictures, to visualize accurately and abstractly
Bodily-kinesthetic intelligence "Body smart"	Ability to control one's body movements and to handle objects skillfully
Musical intelligence "Music smart"	Ability to produce and appreciate rhythm, pitch, and timber
Interpersonal intelligence "People smart"	Capacity to detect and respond appropriately to the moods, motivations, and desires of others
Intrapersonal intelligence "Self smart"	Capacity to be self-aware and in tune with inner feelings, values, beliefs, and thinking processes
Naturalist intelligence "Nature smart"	Ability to recognize and categorize plants, animals, and other objects in nature
Existential intelligence	Sensitivity and capacity to tackle deep questions about human existence such as what is the meaning of life? Why do we die? How did we get here?

Source: Armstrong (n.d.), p. 1.

Once again, if the preferences or intelligences are considered for each individual and the teaching method is tailored to that individual's preference or strength, learning should occur naturally. As it was with the art of passing along knowledge, the science of passing along knowledge is based on appealing to the audience. The use of these models is simply a formalized way of doing so. "If you're thinking about teaching sculpture, I'm not sure that long tracts of verbal descriptions of statues or of sculptures would be a particularly effective way for individuals to learn about works of art. Naturally, these are physical objects and you need to take a look at them, you might even need to handle them" (Cerbin, 2011, 7:45–8:30).

GENERATIONAL DIFFERENCES AND KNOWLEDGE TRANSFER

Think of the earlier description of the relay team's baton handoff. The gap between the runners that is being bridged is a visual that can be compared to the generation gap that must be bridged for the knowledge to be passed. Core values, terminology, and even attention span can vary greatly from generation to generation. There will always be flaws that exist when attempting to apply sweeping generalizations to any group of people. However, the mere exercise of looking at possible differences, the identification of other possible differences, and attempts to identify any misconceptions should lead to a more thoughtful and thus more successful exchange of information. Table 5.2 includes some of the common generalizations that exist regarding the current generations.

TABLE 5.2: GENERATIONAL GENERALIZATIONS

	Silent (1922–1945)	Baby Boomers (1946–1964)	Generation X (1965–1980)	Generation Y/ Millennials (1981–2000)
Historical Event	Great Depression	Vietnam War	Iraq War	September 11
Description	Experienced	Idealistic and competitive	Skeptical and independent	Realistic and collaborative
Work is…	An obligation	An adventure	A contract	A means to an end
Motivator	Security/being respected	Money/being valued	Time off/ freedom and removal of rules	Time off and working with other bright people
Leadership Style	Directive	Quality	Challenges others/asks why	Not yet identified
Work Ethic	Respects authority Works hard Age = Seniority	Workaholics Desires quality Questions authority	Self-reliant Wants structure and direction Skeptical	What's next? Multitasking Tenacity Entrepreneurial
Communication Style	Formal memo	In person	Direct, immediate	Email, voice mail
Technology Event	Hoover Dam	Microwaves	What you can hold in your hand; PDA, cell phone	Ethereal - intangible

Stance on Work–Life Balance	Keep work and life separate	No balance, "live to work"	Balance "work to live"	Balance: It's 5 pm; I have another gig
Money is…	My livelihood	A status symbol	A means to an end	Today's payoff
Value	Family/ community	Success	Time	Individuality

Source: Strauss & Howe, 1997.

Knowing the three main theories of the traditional approaches to learning as well as having an understanding of the generational differences enable us to begin to build the bridge between the mentor and the mentee. According to Tanner and Allen (2004), "How students characterize their learning style and with which framework they characterize it might not even be so critically important, although it could contribute to their academic success by promoting self-awareness and the use of learning strategies that work for their learning style" (p. 201). There is no better or worse; there is merely a difference in styles. So, when you're seeking out and receiving knowledge from older generations, you must actively reach.

"Do not then train a child to learning by force and harshness, but direct them to it by what amuses their minds so that you may be better able to discover with accuracy the peculiar bent of the genius of each."

—Plato

Younger generations cannot assume that the older generation will know how to reach out and pass along the experience that they have had any more than the older generation can assume that the younger generations will find their knowledge useful in the future. However, all generations must make the leap of faith that there is value in the sharing of information and human experience. The act of learning is one of active participation rather than passive acceptance of information. By using the knowledge gained regarding learning styles and the generation gap, we should be able to develop guidelines in sharing and accepting knowledge with and from others.

INFORMATION, KNOWLEDGE, WISDOM, AND INSIGHT

In the prior section, the art and science of knowledge receiving was discussed. We touched on terms such as information and knowledge, but we need to explore these terms a little more. This is where some of those generational differences start to become more noticeable.

INFORMATION

Information is defined as data that is:

1. Accurate and timely

2. Specific and organized for a purpose

3. Presented within a context that gives it meaning and relevance

   and

4. Can lead to increased understanding and a decrease in uncertainty (Businessdictionary.com, n.d.)

Information can be thought of as either concrete or ambiguous. *Concrete information* pertains to actuals and realities, whereas *abstract* or *conceptual information* is open to interpretation. For instance, concrete data is your nursing department's monthly budget numbers. Abstract information is conceptual, such as thoughts or ideas, and usually without physical existence. Caring is conceptual—many patients experience it and define it in their own way, yet it is really hard to measure. Concrete information includes facts and data, and ambiguous information includes wisdom and insight. In order to pass and receive knowledge or information between generations, we need to understand these differences in information.

KNOWLEDGE AND WISDOM

Quite often, people equate experience—in terms of the number of years doing something—with great knowledge and wisdom. However, knowledge and wisdom are two very different concepts, even between cultures. *Knowledge* is the accumulation of facts and data (concrete facts) as well as concepts (abstract information) you have learned or experienced. This would include learning how to create a departmental budget from your mentor. *Wisdom* is the ability to discern and judge which aspects of that knowledge are true, right, lasting, and applicable to your life (Scuderi, n.d.).

INSIGHT

Have you ever had an "a-ha!" moment? An a-ha is a moment of sudden insight or discovery (Oxford online dictionary, n.d.). We have all had (or we should all have had at least once in our lives) a moment of sudden understanding of something we did not understand or comprehend. *Insight* is the deepest level of knowing and the most meaningful to an individual's own life and the awareness of the underlying essence of a truth (Scuderi, n.d.). Insight is the ability to know when you might change or apply the knowledge gained from your mentor to your own life. Many memorable a-ha moments for nurses occur within the first year after

O---▶

"The worst pain a man can suffer: to have insight into much and power over nothing."
–Herodotus

graduating from nursing school. Suddenly, knowledge that was given to you makes sense as you start to practice nursing independently.

INFORMATION AND KNOWLEDGE OVER TIME

It is also important to acknowledge that a large amount of our facts and data can change over time. Knowledge is about facts that we all acquire through our own experiences (Scuderi, 2015). Although things such as generally accepted accounting principles have remained relatively the same, many things have not. In addition, we develop so much new knowledge each day that even what knowledge we hold important can change moment to moment.

Consider this—in 2012, each *minute* saw the following (imagine what these numbers would look like today!):

- 571 new websites were created.
- Twitter users sent 100,000 tweets.
- Facebook users shared 684,478 pieces of content.
- Email users sent 204,166,667 messages.
- YouTube users uploaded 48 hours of new videos.
- The mobile web received 217 new users.
- WordPress users published 347 new blogs.
- Apple received about 47,000 app downloads (James, 2012).

In addition, in 2010, the knowledge being created every 2 days was as much as the knowledge we created from the dawn of civilization up until 2003 (Siegler, 2010). With the explosion of the Internet, information is everywhere. Even more important is that knowledge is not held by any one person or entity.

WISDOM AND INSIGHT BETWEEN GENERATIONS

Both professional nursing organizations and state boards of nursing expect all nurses, from staff nurses to managers to executives, to practice nursing from a base with sufficient evidence. Although each of us might believe that we are experts in our areas, we also must understand that expert opinion is valid, but it is also the lowest form of accepted knowledge on an evidence-based practice (EBP) pyramid, or knowledge hierarchy. Instead of imposing expert opinion, or your knowledge, onto others, maybe the better value is to share wisdom and insight, which is more applicable than expert opinion of the knowledge and data you hold.

> *"There is nothing so terrible as activity without insight."*
> *—Johann Wolfgang von Goethe*

The quote by Johann Wolfgang von Goethe on this page is a good example of how nurses can become so busy, we do not spend the time reflecting on our actions. As we receive mentorship, do we spend the time to reflect on the wisdom and insight or just consider it knowledge for another day? As the baby boomers retire, how do they pass on their wisdom and insight to Generation X and Generation Y, and do we take the time to receive it? Based on Generation Y's size, they will make up roughly 75% of the world's workforce by 2025. Generation Z or the Nexters are already entering college and the workforce.

It is vital that each generation understands how to impart and receive information that is based on wisdom and insight to continue to create the best tomorrow for everyone. The following are some basics for every generation to understand:

- No one of us knows everything.

- We can all learn from each other.

129

- We all complement each other.

- We can mentor and be mentored by any generational person.

Additionally, although baby boomers may believe that they are the primary mentors for all generations that follow them, they are mainly the mentors for Generation X. Generation X, in turn, primarily mentors Generation Y. So, if any one of the generations were to impart wisdom and insight to any other, what would that look like? Review the main characteristics of imparting and receiving wisdom as described in Table 5.3 and ask yourself the following questions:

- What wisdom and insight do I want to pass along to another generation?

- In order for that information to be heard, what is the best way for me to do that?

- What are my biases, and am I managing them in my communication?

- Am I giving my mentor full attention and taking the time to reflect to build my own wisdom and insight?

TABLE 5.3: GENERATIONAL PERSPECTIVES FOR INFORMATION SHARING

Generation	Generational Perspective for Information Sharing	Preferred Delivery Method for Information Sharing
Silent Generation	Tend not to offer opinions without being asked; great at in-person communication	Face-to-face communication; great storytellers

Baby Boomer	Believe their way is the best way and will expect others to follow that way; respect the effort it took for them to get where they are at	Documented and organized; prefers meetings
Generation X	Strive for feedback but will offer feedback in return; wary of authority, authority means little; very independent and would rather do things independently; hate to be micromanaged; do not "preach" hard work	Manages between phone and email; appreciate their work-life balance
Generation Y	Polite to "authority" but expected that everyone is treated equally; appreciate their unique qualities; impart knowledge in small chunks (add hyperlinks or YouTube videos if you can!)	Prefer text-based communication (messaging, texting, and email) but encourage face-to-face communication to improve skill; have them mentor for improving technology skills in others

As many nurses change roles in the next 25 years, whether through retirement or moving up in the workplace, it is important that each generation reflects on their own wisdom and insight to pass along, not just those generations before them. Each nurse is in a role to mentor, to pass along the wisdom and insight that we gain along our careers and professional paths. While holding knowledge may be a source of individual power for someone, the nursing profession gains nothing if we do not share our knowledge, wisdom, and insight.

ESTABLISHING A MENTORING RELATIONSHIP

I have found establishing mentor relationships to be extremely important in my career. I would say, in fact, that I would not be where I am today without the key mentors in my life. I have had some mentor relationships develop organically when neither I nor my mentor was looking; I have had some people seek me out who saw something in me and wanted to be a part of my career; and I have had mentors who I have sought out because of something I saw in them that I recognized as a quality that I needed to grow in myself. In all of these cases, there has been a personality connection as well—which could be characterized as a professional chemistry, of sorts—and that has always developed into a genuine and mutual care for one another and our professional pursuits. I can also attest to the fact that, regardless of how the mentor relationship is started, both people involved grew in ways they did not expect to grow.

I think it is incredibly important to always be ready and open to a new relationship. This starts with always knowing you have more to learn. The moment we feel we have everything figured out is the moment we close ourselves off to the world around us and miss out on the important experiences and information held by those who came before us.

Overcoming intimidation of people in formal management or leadership positions above us is probably one of the biggest challenges I hear of from my generational cohort, and it's a challenge I have experienced myself. It is worth noting that every time I have been vulnerable and asked someone to help mentor me, the person has been genuinely flattered and sometimes confused or even shocked by my interest.

My best example of overcoming intimidation is when I first started in a manager role after moving to Denver, Colorado. I had left Chicago, Illinois, where I had an exceptional mentor, and I found myself struggling in a new role in a new hospital in a new city. We had some instability in the CNO role at the time, and I was finding it very challenging to navigate in the environment. I felt like I was struggling with communication and feeling very insecure in my role.

About a year into my time there, I was placed on a committee that put me in contact with a woman who was in the VP of quality role. I enjoyed learning from her in these meetings, and I admired her ability to articulate her needs and concerns to the group in a way that was heard and respected; she had the very skill I was trying to develop at the time. She had been in the organization a long time, so I knew she was stable there, which was comforting in the time of instability in our CNO office. She and I had a good personal connection, and I genuinely enjoyed learning from her and watching her work.

So, despite my insecurity and embarrassment, I took the opportunity to ask her one day if she and I could have lunch. I explained I saw many qualities in her that I wanted to develop in myself, and I asked if she would be interested in mentoring me.

To my surprise, she was caught off guard and humbled by my request. She was more than willing to do this and was very appreciative that I had said something to her. Soon we were meeting monthly for formal meetings to process through work situations and to develop strategies for me to further my success in the organization. That was 7 years ago, and both she and I have gone through many transitions in the organization. She is now the acting CEO, and I am one of the senior directors in nursing. Through these 7 years, we have continued to meet as a professional need arises, but we also now meet up more regularly as trusted colleagues. Today we have much more of a reciprocal relationship, and we go to each other with concerns or questions or just when we need help. I am so glad I was courageous enough to approach her 7 years ago, as I have learned so much about my own career and I have also learned how to be a mentor to those who come across my path.

—Amy Brown, MS, RN, NE-BC

As a parent, I want my children to exceed what I have accomplished in life, and I want them to do it more easily and faster if possible. I would ask the same of any generation mentoring the next. If you expect the generations after you to work as hard and as long as you did, or accomplish things the same way you accomplished things, ask yourself why? What do you get from holding back mentorship, holding back help or insight, by slowing the growth of others in order to see them accomplish things the same way you did? If the benefit is to help your ego, then consider that maybe you are not suited to be a mentor. But if you want to mentor others, allow them to do things their own way, building from your insight and wisdom, then help them understand what needs to live on and what is okay to go away. For those who belong to Generations X and Y, what do you need to learn to take over most management positions in the next 10 years? The success of our profession and the health of our population depend on our professional and personal growth.

A WEALTH OF KNOWLEDGE

We are bombarded with data on a minute-by-minute basis. Data is individual pieces of information such as "facts, numbers, letters and symbols that describe an object, situation, or other factors" (National Academies Press, 1999, p. 15). Text messaging, email, and smartphone applications that keep us updated on everything from world events to the latest clothing sales are all examples of data being pushed to us in a constant barrage of dings and beeps. The amount of electronic data is so large it is now measured in exabytes (the prefix *exa* means 1 billion billion).

> *"He uses statistics as a drunken man uses lamp-posts…for support rather than illumination."*
> –Andrew Lang

Information is data that is useful and can provide answers to "who, what, where, and when" questions (Ackoff, 1989). Much of the data we produce can provide an extraordinary amount of information, if we know how to use it.

This extraordinary amount of data also has led to an information obsession with staying up to date on the latest trends, stock markets, and clinical practices halfway around the world. Whatever you want to know about, you can have access to in a few seconds time. The following passage by Reed (2010) points to the positives of what would otherwise be an overload:

> Everywhere you look, the quantity of information in
> the world is soaring. Merely keeping up with this flood,
> and storing the bits that might be useful, is difficult
> enough. Analyzing it, to spot patterns and extract use-
> ful information, is harder still. Even so, the data deluge
> is already starting to transform business, government,
> science and everyday life...It has great potential for
> good—as long as consumers, companies, and govern-
> ments make the right choices about when to restrict
> the flow of data, and when to encourage it (pp. 10–12).

This obsession takes time. It also takes energy. To make the most of your time, you need to know what is just data, just information, and then what knowledge is. Knowledge is the appropriate collection of information intended to be useful (Ackoff, 1989). How do we keep up with all of the information that is available to us without losing sight of the fact that having knowledge and knowing what to do with that knowledge are two very different things? We begin by learning to recognize value.

It has been said that getting information off the Internet is like taking a drink from a fire hose. Christopher J. Frank and Paul Magnone (2011) wrote a book aptly named *Drinking from the Fire Hose*, which has been hailed as a game changer in the data management world. In the book the pair outlines seven questions, described in Table 5.4, to sort through mass quantities of data and identify the information that will help you make better business decisions.

TABLE 5.4: THE SEVEN QUESTIONS FROM *DRINKING FROM THE FIRE HOSE*

Question	Action
What is the essential business question?	Asking the right question is the key to finding the indispensable answer in the mountain of information.
Where is your customer's North Star?	Shift your view from company-centric to customer-centric.
Should you believe the squiggly line?	Question the validity of short-term data.
What surprised you?	Uncover hidden information and use it to change the dialogue.
What does the Lighthouse reveal?	Identify the risks, barriers, and bridges that surround your business.
Who are your swing voters?	Drive growth, increase revenue, and boost satisfaction by looking at your existing customer in a new way.
What? So what? Now what?	Follow this easy-to-remember sequence of questions to effectively communicate results and inspire action.

Source: Frank and Magnone, 2011.

Although Frank and Magnone constructed the book and the Seven Questions with a business perspective in mind, their application is much broader. Nurse leaders can use these questions to dig into clinical and financial data and ferret out whether the data in general is even useful. The questions force you to gain a new perspective regarding information. They cut through what is commonly referred to as *analysis paralysis*. The Seven Questions shift the focus from the data, which is merely historical information, to a forward-thinking, action-based discussion or thought process.

The Seven Questions also shift us away from the traditional methods utilized in formal education that lead us to believe that whoever has the longest slide presentation or the most complicated graph has mastered the concept being taught in that course or presented in the boardroom. In contrast, the new test of mastering a skill or concept would then be the boiling down of all knowledge gained to its simplest and most applicable form. The seventh question (What? So what? Now what?) leads us to an objectivity untainted with the time it took to collect the data or money paid to be in the class. If it is not applicable and able to be used to do something…so what? It is this discernment that will need to be applied if we are to have enough energy left to act and keep up with the exabytes that will inevitably keep coming.

THE VALUE OF KNOWLEDGE

The belief that knowledge has an inherent value dates back to the first century, when Juvenal (55–130) stated, "All wish to know, but none wish to pay the price." The invention and wide usage of the Internet and smartphones have created a point where a mass amount of knowledge is accessible to the public, for nearly no cost. Up until this last decade, the encyclopedia, which has been around for more than 2,000 years, was used to provide a general, but comprehensive, summary of all knowledge.

So, why is this important? Anyone can get the knowledge you hold, and they can possibly even get it for free. What they cannot necessarily get, though, is the wisdom and insight that comes along with it. Wisdom and insight have an intrinsic value; their value can be regarded as an end in itself.

IS THE INFORMATION RELEVANT?

In all doctoral programs, you drink from that fire hydrant of information. In my PhD program, this fire hydrant specifically spewed peer-reviewed articles and book chapters. Although the expectation was that I would read everything, not everything was interesting, and not all of it made sense in the larger scheme of things at the time I was reading it. Granted, I attempted to read the information, but I would set it in the pile to be kept for a time at which I might find it helpful. Now, I am glad that I had the insight at that time to save all the articles and books we were supposed to read. I printed everything and had binders for all the courses. Many articles were highlighted in many different color markers; others had no markups or notes. However, when my formal classes were done, and I was studying for my comprehensive exams, I found those articles that were not highlighted to be some of the most helpful articles. As I read them, I was surprised that it seemed like I was reading them for the first time. When I had previously read them, I had not acknowledged, or I had not had the ability to acknowledge, the relevance of the information I was receiving.

WHAT IS VALUABLE AND WHAT IS NOT

As noted earlier, there is an amazing amount of knowledge being created daily from all the data and information available. For a decision about staffing on a medical unit in a hospital, there may be more tools available today, but there is also more knowledge governing that decision. Remember, not all knowledge is useful, particularly if the receiver of the information does not see it as knowledge, but only as information. Sometimes what one considers knowledge might never be useful to someone regardless, whereas at another time and place it might be.

Sometimes, there is no best time to give someone information, and no best time to receive information. I have students today who ask why they did not get a certain article sooner or learn about one subject before another subject. I liken it to answering the question, "Which came first—the chicken or the egg?" There is no right answer, so it depends on each of us to give knowledge and to receive it at any time. For those of us receiving knowledge, if it does not make sense, tuck it away for later. Remember—respect the people who are giving you the information because it has a meaning for them and they want to share it. It is up to you ultimately to use it and to have insight on its larger application for you.

Tips for receiving information, knowledge, wisdom, and insight:

- Listen to understand what information you are being told.

- Ask the person giving you this information as many questions as it takes so that you understand what the person is trying to impart to you.

- Be thankful for the information; the person passing it to you felt that you were worth telling.

- Hold on to information that might not be immediately usable; all information has some value even though you might not immediately recognize its value.

- Recognize that the information you are being given has some meaning to the person who is delivering it to you.

- Keep track of yourself; in other words, be open and appreciative of information you are getting. Do not become flippant, arrogant, or dismissive, which would only demonstrate to others you are not open to communication.

By recognizing that all information has some value or meaning to someone, you will help create a supportive, positive environment for everyone—those who are giving the information, and those who are receiving it.

COMMON GROUND

Common ground can be either a physical space or a conceptual space where individuals recognize commonalities and can speak as well as listen. And although it might seem, given all the generational differences, that finding common ground for the transfer of knowledge would be difficult, it is not—*nursing* is our common ground! Each generation of nurses wants to know that they made a difference, that patients' lives improved through contact with them, and that the profession became stronger.

In organizations where mentoring is a formal process—where an individual seeks out another or is assigned to another individual—the need to find common ground might not be as critical. The mere fact that formal mentoring is occurring might be the common ground.

FINDING COMMON GROUND

If the mentoring is not formal, or arranged, you should always work to achieve common ground. There are formal methods and steps to determine common ground. One method for determining common ground is through *Rogerian argument*, a strategy in which participants collaborate to find areas of shared experience (Baumlin, 1987). This method of reasoning attempts to find a compromise between two sides unlike each other, which are more adversarial, seeking to find the one winner. To practice this method, there are four stages, which are described in the following list. Although the stages speak to written communication, you can instead use these steps for a script for a meeting.

1. An introduction to the problem and a demonstration that the opponent's position is understood.

2. A statement of the contexts in which the opponent's position may be valid.

3. A statement of the writer's position, including the contexts in which it is valid.

4. A statement of how the opponent's position would benefit if he were to adopt elements of the writer's position. If the writer can show that the positions complement each other, that each supplies what the other lacks, so much the better (Young, Becker, & Pike, 1970, p. 283).

There may be variations to the Rogerian method, but the key point is that an individual must be able to state the opposing viewpoint first—before stating his own—with honesty, with understanding, and without overt or covert evaluation (Brent, 1996). Through this process, you may still not agree with the opposing point of view, but you will have an empathetic perspective. In restating another's position, you will start to learn the person's underlying belief (Brent). Through understanding this underlying belief, common ground can be determined, and the successful passing and receiving of knowledge can be achieved.

KNOWING WHEN TO RESIST AND WHEN TO GIVE UP

For those who have never heard this saying, it is about not choosing a battle that's not worth winning. With different generations in the workplace, conflicts will occur. Conflicts might even occur between you and your mentor/mentee. For many of us, our personality type (as described earlier) guides how we decide to not give up or to let something go. Whichever way you choose, remember you have a lot of control over giving up or letting something go and the ultimate outcome. However, you have to use wisdom and insight to make the right decision. It is never easy to walk away, but this should not mean you were wrong. This is particularly hard for those of us in Generations X and Y because we strive to be seen as independent and "good enough." Those qualities do not mean you will win every battle—nor should you. Your worth is not less if you back down.

IS IT WORTH THE FIGHT?

If you are going to die on the proverbial hill, first ask yourself these questions (Haggard, 2010):

> Do you understand the real problem?
>
> Is what you are trying to accomplish under your control?
>
> Is it worth the time and effort?
>
> Will you remember this a year from now?
>
> Are the consequences of losing worth the battle?
>
> Are the consequences of winning worth the battle?

If you answer no to any of these, take time to reflect and decide on your next steps. Learn how to gracefully give up on something that was not meant to be; don't fight just because you feel you have been challenged.

PERSONAL APPLICATION

The following questions are designed to help you reflect on the knowledge and wisdom you have gained over your career and to facilitate the successful transfer of this knowledge and wisdom to those nurse leaders who, like you, have devoted their life's work to their patients and to the nursing profession.

1. Personality plays a role in passing and receiving information.

    - What personality tests have you taken? At minimum, take the Myers-Briggs Type Indicator (http://www.myersbriggs.org).

    - How does what you understand about your personality have an impact on how you hand off information? How you receive information?

2. Acknowledging differences in learning styles (visual, aural, reading/writing, and/or kinesthetic) is key to successful knowledge and wisdom transfer.

    - How does your preferred learning style influence how you take and give information?

    - Can you recognize the preferred learning style of your mentor/mentee or colleagues?

    - How will you complement your learning style with others in order to effectively receive and/or pass on knowledge, wisdom, and insight?

3. Being an introvert or extrovert can influence your perception of and relationship with others.

    - Are you an extrovert or an introvert?

    - Who among the individuals you work with are introverts? Extroverts?

    - How will you change the way you work with both so that you can maximize the mentoring relationship?

4. Every individual identifies with one of the nine types of intelligences.

    - What is your preferred intellectual ability?

    - How do you use that intelligence within your mentoring?

- What is the intelligence type of the person whom you are mentoring/being mentored by?
- Do you tailor your preferred type to relate to another's unique aptitude and set of capabilities?

5. Knowledge, wisdom, and insight are in some ways similar but they have distinct meanings.

- Do you reflect on the information you are giving someone in a mentoring relationship?
- Is this information good for the here and now, or will it be useful over the mentee's career?

6. In order to work together effectively and successfully, all generations need to find common ground.

- When you differ on a topic, instead of blaming a generational difference, do you explore or find common ground before proceeding?
- What does that common ground look like?

LOOKING FORWARD

For younger generations, it is important to be ready to receive knowledge from older generations. This readiness includes being open to information and others' ideas, opinions, and perspectives. Not all information you receive may be welcome or even immediately useful. It is important to ensure respectful and open lines of communication with others so that you can learn from everyone. Everyone from every generation has knowledge, experience, and wisdom to share. Although learning can occur between any generations, the younger generations must listen and empathize in order to learn what may be applicable now and what might be applicable later.

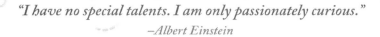

"I have no special talents. I am only passionately curious."
—*Albert Einstein*

6

STRATEGIES FOR SUCCESSFUL KNOWLEDGE & WISDOM TRANSFER

AMY STEINBINDER, PHD, RN, NE-BC
JANICE GANANN, MED, PCC

CHAPTER OBJECTIVES

Explain how curiosity, inquisitiveness, and being a student of nurse colleagues' experiences leads to understanding, appreciation, and ability to apply what was learned to one's own career.

Identify the roles and benefits of mentoring and ways to establish an effective mentoring relationship.

Describe ways that the power of collaboration can support accomplishing significant goals.

The premise of this chapter is based on the belief that when we create meaningful relationships, we are poised to seamlessly transfer wisdom and are able to achieve our personal and professional goals faster, with fewer false starts, and with a greater sense of purpose, clarity, satisfaction, and accomplishment. At the same time, we are also contributing to the profession and/or science of nursing. As we address workforce transitions, those individuals leaving and others stepping into the roles that have been vacated, the impact and value of meaningful relationships become increasingly important. In this chapter, we identify and describe six strategies that foster the development of these significant relationships. We begin, however, by defining what a relationship is as it pertains to knowledge transfer.

RELATIONSHIPS IN THE CONTEXT OF KNOWLEDGE TRANSFER

The definition of *relationship* is broad and has several meanings. For the purposes of this chapter, a *relationship* encompasses connecting, associating, or being involved with another person for the purpose of creating strong bonds (The Free Dictionary, n.d.). These strong bonds are formed to accomplish specific goals, tasks, or purposes and may be either informal or formal.

It's important to consider, from the perspectives of both nurse professionals—the retiring nurse executive and the early-career nurse—what connects or binds each party in the relationship:

- What is each giving up and/or gaining?
- What does each participant want/need from the other party?

- How can each ensure that individual needs and expectations are addressed?

It's also important to identify the elements that create an effective, trusting relationship. We used the following assumptions to guide the development of this chapter:

- The retiring nurse professional has something to share and contribute to the profession of nursing, the discipline, and often to the organization.

- The receiving nurse professional is interested in learning what is being shared/contributed.

- Personal relationships provide greater opportunity for sharing wisdom than what can be gleaned from academic/formal learning.

- There is no substitute for experience.

- Opening doors for those receiving information creates awareness for them regarding the current state of their knowledge—"I don't know what I don't know."

STRATEGIES FOR KNOWLEDGE TRANSFER

We have identified six strategies to support the development of relationships for the purposes of supporting integration across the generations. The six strategies are as follows:

1. Storytelling

2. Mentoring process

3. Powerful questions

4. Career planning

5. Collaboration and wisdom sharing

6. Recognizing and celebrating

In the following sections we describe each of these relationship strategies in detail.

STORYTELLING

Most common wisdom in organizations is passed on through storytelling. A story is a description of what happened in a situation. Storytelling also conveys the values of an organization, reveals the culture, explains how people are rewarded, and describes how people work. Stories provide the emotional context for a situation and are powerful tools in human growth and development.

"It is the heart always that sees, before the head can see."
—Thomas Carlyle

Over the past few years, there has been an ongoing interest in storytelling as a component of knowledge management. Storytelling has been touted as one of the best ways to make the leap from information to knowledge, and is recommended as the best way to capture and transfer tacit knowledge. Sole and Wilson (2002) report that sharing experiences through stories cultivates trust, allows us to transfer our tacit knowledge, establishes emotional connections, and even facilitates unlearning.

Stories help us appreciate where we have been and position us to explore the future. Storytelling is a traditional—even ancient—means of passing on wisdom and culture. Although there are a variety of strategies for conveying knowledge within organizations—including mentoring; apprenticeships; experiential simulation; coded resources, such as manuals and textbooks; and maps, symbols, and illustrations—storytelling is an excellent strategy for conveying norms and values, building trust and commitment, preparing for change, and generating the emotional connections necessary to share knowledge.

PERSONAL GROWTH

Early in my career, I was responsible for coordinating a continuing education conference. The marketing brochure was drafted. I had spent hours creating it and reviewing it. When I thought it was ready, I sent the brochure to the printer. When the brochure was delivered from the print shop, there was a typographical error. I was mortified—and I was certain I was going to be fired.

When my boss called me into her office, she said, "What have you learned from this experience?" I stated that I would have multiple people, preferably individuals who had not been involved in the planning process, review any document prior to sending any marketing materials to the printers. And then I shared with her that I thought I was going to be fired. Her response was, "Why would I fire you? I've just made a significant investment in your development!"

The lesson learned was powerful. I felt valued by my supervisor. We are all human, and we all make mistakes. People learn and grow from their mistakes, and I had established a process to mitigate this type of mistake in the future.

—Amy Steinbinder, PhD, RN, NE-BC

What stories do you want to tell? Think of those experiences that had a strong effect on your career. Those "ah-ha" moments that—now that you reflect back on them—were transformational to you early in your career. How can you provide the story that captures your insights and learnings to share with others?

MENTORING

A *mentor* is an experienced professional; a *mentee* is a less-experienced one. Successful people often have had one or more mentors in their career. Mentors offer advice on what to do, how to do it, and why something is worth doing in a situation. Ideally, mentors and mentees self-select each other and use structure and tools to support their learning.

Healthcare is an increasingly complex and challenging industry that demands well-qualified, prepared, innovative, and dynamic individuals to lead organizations and people into the future. One method for better preparing future leaders is establishing a formal mentoring program to allow early-career nurses to partner with senior-level leaders.

> *"I am always doing that which I cannot do, in order that I may learn how to do it."*
> *—Pablo Picasso*

REFLECTIONS FROM A NURSE LEADER

Rhonda Anderson, DNSc, RN, FAAN, FACHE, CEO of Banner Cardon Children's Medical Center, states, "Mentoring is providing opportunities for a young professional to be seen and to encourage them to be agile, trusted professionals and leaders." Anderson has mentored many individuals throughout her career, and she shares four principles that guide her mentoring relationships:

- **Availability.** "The young professionals I am mentoring can call, text, or stop by my office anytime they need me," says Anderson.

- **Notes of encouragement.** "As we are learning and growing, knowing that someone believes in us is important. I want them to know I believe in them," says Anderson. When possible, this means adding the personal touch of writing a note and sending it in the mail, rather than typing an email (although Anderson does that, too).

- **Literature of interest.** "If I find an article about an area of interest of theirs, I will forward it to them," says Anderson.

- **Maintaining constant contact.** "It is important to continue the relationships, even after the formal mentoring has concluded. I maintain contact with many individuals who have gone on to become chief nursing officers and chief executive officers of hospitals and other healthcare organizations today," says Anderson.

Another key tenet to mentoring, Anderson explains, is understanding an individual's core values. Knowing who that individual is and what that individual holds important promotes a stronger, trusting relationship. Anderson's job as the mentor is to "fill in new learning." She fondly recalls her mentor, June Werner, MN, MSN, RN, CNAA, who received the Creative Nursing Magazine Mentor award in 1995: "She was such an amazing human being and had a profound impact on my life and career." As a result, Anderson has given back to the nursing profession. She is actively involved in the mentoring programs for Global Nursing Exchange, American Organization of Nurse Executives (AONE), and American College of Healthcare Executives (ACHE) (R. Anderson, personal communication, May 25, 2015).

In addition, the more structured a mentoring program for creating knowledge transfer is, the better. Determine the early-career nurse's goals and developmental needs, and then pair that individual with a more experienced nurse leader to create cross-organizational dialogue among generations. There are various mentoring models, including one-on-one sessions, group programs, senior leadership discussion panels, or "speed mentoring" programs (where nurses sit across from organizational experts to ask questions). No matter what method you choose, making mentoring a part of the relationships you establish with early-career nurses will ensure that the organization's history and knowledge continue from one generation to the next.

As Anderson shares, being a mentor provided as much reward and fulfillment to her as it did to those she was mentoring. It's a way to recharge your batteries, keep you engaged, and grow while assisting others to fulfill their professional aspirations.

HOW MENTORING RELATIONSHIPS WORK

Mentoring is designed to offer the mentee development opportunities, career advice, and an opportunity to learn from a more senior person who is reflecting on experiences that the mentor has gained. The mentor and mentee must be mutually committed to a beneficial relationship, which requires honesty, openness, dedication, and effort. Also, the mentor and mentee must be responsible with confidential or proprietary information.

MENTORING

Kunich and Lester (1999) provide the following mnemonic—using the term *MENTORING*—to help you remember the actions that will strengthen the mentoring experience:

M	Model
E	Empathize
N	Nurture
T	Teach
O	Organize
R	Respond
I	Inspire
N	Network
G	Goal Set

Steve Trautman (2014), a recognized author and speaker on the subject of knowledge transfer, recommends addressing the following four crucial questions to successfully mentor peers:

- **Whom do you want to teach?** Experts need a clearly assigned apprentice. And, the apprentice needs to know that learning from the expert is a job expectation for which the apprentice is accountable.

- **What do you want me to teach?** Experts and apprentices need to know, down to the task level, what is high-priority knowledge to be transferred.

- **When should I teach and transfer this knowledge?** Set a clear amount of time to be spent on knowledge transfer.

- **How should I teach so that the mentee gets it quickly and correctly?** Some experts are naturals at sharing their knowledge, but there are also those who are not. Provide tools and techniques for good knowledge transfer, such as how to write a clear agenda and what questions to ask to ensure knowledge was absorbed and retained.

Those individuals in the mentor role have specific responsibilities:

- Identify goals and objectives.

- Define and establish a plan.

- Meet regularly for dialogue and to discuss progress.

- Commit to a 1-year relationship (which may be extended).

- Inculcate the mentee into the organizational culture.

- Introduce the mentee to people in the organization and transition key relationships.

- Listen and offer feedback.

- Communicate experiences and challenges.

As a result of mentoring, mentors gain new perspectives, learn new information, refine their coaching and feedback skills, and gain personal satisfaction by helping someone develop.

Those individuals in the mentee role also have specific responsibilities:

- Identify goals and objectives.

- Ask questions and inquire.

- Listen.

- Share information openly about career goals and needs.

- Be open to feedback from the mentor.

- Demonstrate progress toward goal attainment.

Benefits for the mentee include expanded networks and greater visibility, career guidance, personal growth, and insight from a leader with different experiences than the mentee.

To better facilitate the identification of shared goals in the mentoring relationship, individuals in the mentor role will find it helpful to develop a shared goals worksheet like the one shown in Figure 6.1.

LEADERSHIP MENTORING: SHARED GOALS

Objectives	Discussion	Action or Follow-Up
Session 1 1. Establish the goals for the mentoring relationships. 2. Identify your strengths, passions, and areas of expertise.	What are your career goals? Where do you want to be in 3–5 years? What will it take for you to be successful?	Create a vision statement for where you want to be in 3–5 years. Identify the skills needed to obtain that position.
Session 2 1. Learn how to create an annual department budget.	Financial management has been identified as an area of development.	Provide introduction to Susan Brown, cost-accounting resource in finance department.
Session 3		
Session 4		

Figure 6.1   Sample Shared Goals Worksheet

Formal mentoring helps build leaders for the future and gives mentors an opportunity to invest in and contribute to the organization over the long term. It can lead to the following outcomes:

- Demonstrated professional growth and development

- Evidence of critical thinking related to specific leadership issues

- Identified opportunities for the mentee

- Reported knowledge gain and decision-making capability

- Demonstrated effective leadership behaviors

Although formal mentoring is extremely valuable for ensuring the next generation is learning and growing, the mentoring relationship does not need to be a formal process that's set up or coordinated through your organization, a professional association, or working relationship. If you are an experienced professional, look for someone who is early in his or her career, whom you admire, and who has great potential, and then identify ways you can support and encourage that person. If you are an early-career individual, think about those people whom you admire—

maybe they are in a specific role, have a particular skill, or possess a leadership trait that you appreciate. Seek out those individuals to ask for their support and assistance. Both parties will undoubtedly benefit from the mentoring relationship.

"The final test of a leader is that he leaves behind in other men the conviction and the will to carry on."
—Walter Lippmann

POWERFUL QUESTIONS

Questions have the power to change lives. They can jump-start creativity, change our perspective, empower us to believe in ourselves, push us to think things through, or call us to action. As adults, we learn what we want to learn, when we want to know it. So, as knowledge is transferred and relationships are transitioned, it is important for both parties to be open, to be curious, and to ask questions.

"He who asks is a fool for five minutes, but he who does not ask remains a fool forever."
—Chinese proverb

In their book *Co-Active Coaching*, Kimsey-House et al. (2011) state:

> Curiosity starts with a question. The interesting thing about
> a question is that it automatically causes us to start looking.
> For example, when you read the question, What is the weather
> like today?, chances are you started thinking about the weather
> in your town. We have a Pavlovian response to a question. It
> nearly throws us in the direction of the question, looking for an
> answer.
>
> Our experience in school trained us to gather information by
> asking specific questions that enable us to deduce answers. In
> that environment, we learned that questions have specific an-
> swers—in fact, right answers. Even essay questions have correct
> answers that are specific, concrete, and measurable. We learned
> that questions are used to narrow possibilities. This is the
> deductive method. We learned to fill in the blanks, and
> we learned about being scored on our ability to get the right
> answer.
>
> There is a big difference between conventional questions that
> elicit information and curious questions that evoke personal
> exploration (p. 69–70).

Curiosity is a component of the foundation on which meaningful relationships are built. As Theodore Roosevelt so eloquently stated, "People
don't care how much you know, until they know how much you care." If
we use that premise while transitioning relationships and transferring
knowledge, we will establish solid, trustful relationships with the next
generation. One approach to building these kinds of relationship is quite
simple: Ask questions.

STOP INTERRUPTING!

How long does it take for us to seek to understand what someone is interested in achieving? Studies show that healthcare workers interrupt patients within 17 seconds of them sharing what is going on (Rhoades, McFarland, Finch, & Johnson, 2001; Inskeep & Groopman, 2007). If we do that "in our formal roles," how quickly are we going to interrupt someone we are mentoring? Here's a challenge: Ask someone you care about, or the individual you are mentoring, "What are your personal aspirations?" or "What would you like to achieve in your career?" and don't interrupt them for one full minute. It is amazing what you will hear and learn in that 60 seconds.

Asking questions is relatively easy. Asking the right questions—better questions that we call *powerful questions*—takes a bit more consideration. *Powerful questions* are open-ended questions that require more than a yes or no response. These questions generally begin with words such as *what*, *how*, *when*, and *why*. However, be mindful when using "why" as it can elicit defensiveness—depending on the situation and your nonverbal behavior. When you ask "why?" you might be perceived as scolding or being accusatory.

Why, as leaders, do we not ask better questions? Perhaps it's because we believe that having the right answer is most important. We pride ourselves on our ability to quickly find solutions and fixes. We operate under the assumption that we are paid to fix problems rather than to foster breakthrough learning. Not knowing the answer to a current problem makes most people uncomfortable.

As we are growing and developing the next generation of nurse leaders, our primary role is to foster their learning. One way to expedite the process is by utilizing powerful questions in professional relationships. Senge and his colleagues (1994) promote the use of powerful questions to serve as provocative queries and to expose confusion and evasiveness. By asking the powerful question, clarity, action, and discovery are made possible. As you can see from the examples in the following list, powerful questions are generally short, open-ended questions that create a greater possibility for expanded learning and a fresh perspective:

- What do you want?

- How would you like to contribute to the nursing profession?

- What's another perspective you could take?

- How will you know you've been successful?

Isn't that why we ask questions in the first place—to learn? Don't we strive to always be curious and inquisitive?

CAREER PLANNING

Continuous career planning and skill enhancement are necessities in today's ever-changing healthcare environment. Knowing your strengths, goals, and aspirations is key to creating, managing, and evaluating your career options.

As a seasoned nurse, can you remember your first day on the job? Remember the mixed emotions: how excited you were; how afraid you were of making a mistake or hurting a patient? Now, in hindsight what do you wish you had known or that someone had told you? As you are developing relationships and mentoring the next generation of nurses, the following set of steps may be useful to you as you guide and assist others with planning their career. The worksheet shown in Figure 6.2 will guide your career planning process.

O---▶

"Our chief want is someone who will inspire us to be what we know we could be."

–Ralph Waldo Emerson

CAREER PLANNING

Step 1: Describe your ideal job.

- How will it leverage your strengths and experiences?
- Does it align with your interests and values?
- What is the path to that job?
- What knowledge, skills, competencies, and experiences do you need in order to obtain that job?

Remember: The ideal job might change over time so it is important to reassess values, interests, competencies, and experiences on an annual basis.

Step 2: Create your action plan by setting career goals.

- Think 3–5 years out.
- Set SMART goals:

  Is your goal specific?

  Is your goal measurable?

  Is your goal actionable?

  Is your goal realistic?

  Is your goal timely?

Step 3: Execute the plan.

- Performance drives everything—perform in your current role.
- Focus on competency and/or experience gaps.
- Develop an expertise.
- Be proactive—don't wait on your manager or the organization.
- Be patient and build skills that increase your marketability.

Figure 6.2   Sample Career Planning Worksheet

Career planning is a tool/resource that can be facilitated/co-created between the nurse leader and early-career nurse as they establish a mentoring relationship and as a part of the succession planning process.

Experienced leaders have insights and perspectives that can assist early-career nurses in considering options for the remainder of their careers.

The literature is replete with information and tactical approaches used to address the first four strategies described in this chapter. However, for the next two strategies—"Collaboration and Wisdom Sharing" and "Recognizing and Celebrating"—that is not the case. The power of these last two strategies will be illustrated using the unique and personal stories of two great nurse leaders.

COLLABORATION AND WISDOM SHARING

Collaboration is an essential component of creating meaningful relationships, and it is conducive to sharing our wisdom. Wikipedia (n.d.) defines *collaboration* as "working with others to do a task and to achieve shared goals." The definition elaborates that collaboration is "more than the intersection of common goals seen in co-operative ventures, but a deep, collective determination to reach an identical objective ... by sharing knowledge, learning and building consensus. The result of collaboration is the ability to obtain greater resources, recognition and reward even when in the face of finite resources."

"What we do for ourselves dies with us. What we do for others and the world remains and is immortal."

–Albert Pine

What is possible when one nurse scientist and researcher chooses to share her wisdom by collaborating with other like-minded nurse scientists and researchers? The journey of renowned nurse scientist and researcher Marlene Kramer illustrates the power of collaboration and wisdom sharing. Kramer has dedicated her life's work to gaining understanding and clarity about the work environment of clinical nurses employed in acute care hospitals. In the 1960s, while she served as faculty at the University of California at San Francisco, Kramer became curious about why many clinical nurses experience reality shock whereas others do not. She interviewed clinical nurses who found themselves in need of telling their stories, and in the process they were unburdening themselves of their experiences. She then published *Reality Shock: Why Nurses Leave Nursing* in 1974. Over the years, as Kramer continued to publish, refine, and expand her research, she became the expert on identifying and defining workplace attributes that contributed to empowered professional nursing practice.

Kramer's passion for her research topic, scholarly approach, intriguing findings, and engaging, articulate presentation style led other like-minded scientists to pursue collaborating with Kramer and Kramer's research colleague, Claudia Schmalenberg, to expand research in this area. By the 1990s, Kramer and Schmalenberg had formed Health Science Research Associates (HSRA), a nationally representative group of 23 educators, executives, and researchers in hospitals and professional organizations who work together to study and advance the quality of healthy work environments.

These researchers received no monetary incentives or payment to participate in the research through HSRA; however, they did receive funding through the American Association of Critical-Care Nurses (AACN), and they used the honoraria they received from presenting their research to fund their research travel expenses. Unfortunately, as an entity, they were not eligible to apply for other types of grants. To date, Kramer and her colleagues have collaboratively published 40 studies on the dimensions and essentials of Magnetism, seven reports on 5-year and 7-year studies on healthy practice environments and professional socialization of newly licensed nurses, and an additional three studies on essential professional nursing practices related to effects on patient and nurse outcomes. These studies have contributed greatly to our understanding of the elements of the work environments we have come to know as Magnet environments.

Kramer's attributes of openness, willingness to partner with others, and inclusivity exemplify collaborative wisdom sharing in action. Over the years she has invited other like-minded researchers to join her in her research, which has resulted in a tremendous body of knowledge that likely would not have emerged without her thoughtful, planned approach. Sharing her wisdom and collaborating in many practice environment research studies have made it possible for nurses at all levels to develop and implement practical, evidence-based tactics to improve practice environments and, ultimately, improve patient care.

In preparing for the future, Kramer has relinquished her role as president of HSRA and has passed this important work to two solid researchers who will seamlessly advance the science by conducting robust studies that differentiate outcomes of organizations with healthy work environments and explain the impact of complexity theory on care at the bedside (M. Kramer, personal communication, May 29, 2015).

Ann Van Slyck's journey provides an example of another brilliant, visionary nurse leader, innovator, and entrepreneur. Her leadership career, which began with a traditional role of CNO in the early 1970s, quickly expanded to address a question that had been plaguing nurse executives for some time: How do we acknowledge the unique and significant contributions of clinical nurses, separate nursing care from the bed charge, and shift the mind-set from nursing as a "cost center" to a "revenue producer"? After all, are patients not admitted to hospitals specifically for nursing care regardless of the medical interventions and/or treatments they receive?

In the early '70s, in collaboration with her hospital's executive team, Van Slyck set out to unbundle nursing care from the room and board charge. This work was important to her because she and her colleagues believed that both patients and payers had a right to know what they were purchasing. Up to this time, nursing was the only profession that remained bundled; all other disciplines' services were billed separately. Van Slyck was interested in creating a financial model that could be used to set up the organization for success. Her passion for the finance side of nursing care and patient care delivery led her to establish her own business and continue answering the question, "How can we fiscally quantify the contributions of nurses at the bedside?"

Van Slyck and her company created patient classification (patient acuity determination) to quantify the amount and skill level of nursing care consumed by each patient and to give the hospital the ability to cost, price, and charge for that care. Additionally, they determined an algorithm for predicting patient needs. Hospital CEOs, CFOs, and CNOs wanted the tools Van Slyck and her company developed, and Van Slyck partnered with large IT firms to integrate patient classification (patient acuity determination) into the electronic medical record (EMR). Van Slyck eventually reached a point at which selling her company was the most viable option for taking the company to the next level to provide increasingly robust consulting services and products for hospitals to achieve continued success. Her decision to sell was a difficult one, as her company had been nationally recognized and incorporated for 25 years and had served hospitals in 42 states.

Because Van Slyck's expertise was not in mergers and acquisitions, she and her CFO hired a firm with extensive experience in healthcare mergers and acquisitions. In the 2-year process of looking for a buyer and successfully negotiating the sale, employees of the company were kept apprised of the activities. Based on Van Slyck's past experience, she believed that new owners often terminate existing staff because those individuals signify the old culture, and the new owners try to encourage the new culture to take hold and thrive by hiring new people to replace those who have been terminated. Consequently, in preparation for the sale, Van Slyck downsized the company to minimize the perceived impact of the "culture baggage" (A. Van Slyck, personal communication, May 29, 2015).

Kramer and Van Slyck were always passionate about their science and the creation of thriving organizations. Kramer's consortium of work environment scientists and Van Slyck's multi-million dollar patient classification company resulted in both leaders reflecting on their own areas of expertise and then recognizing how best to serve their respective entities. Both sought out experts to strengthen and grow their science and organization, and they positioned themselves to transition from formal leadership roles into consultative roles as they continued to share their wisdom.

PRINCIPLES OF COLLABORATION AND WISDOM SHARING

The following principles emerged from the interviews of these leaders and were consistent in both cases, despite both women having very different professional trajectories:

- **Follow your passion and vision for a defined area of practice.**
  Both Kramer and Van Slyck had a passion to advance the quality of the healthcare work environment for hospital-based clinical nurses. In Van Slyck's case, her passion was creating business tools to assist hospital leadership teams in determining patient acuity and quantifying the cost, price, and value of nursing care at the bedside. In Kramer's case, her passion was to provide evidence of practice environment attributes for use by nurses at all levels to improve the settings.

- **Create a community of like-minded colleagues.** Both Kramer and Van Slyck organized the work to be done in ways that would be valuable and sustainable. Kramer, in concert with her primary collaborator, created the HSRA consortium. Van Slyck created and incorporated Van Slyck and Associates.

- **Meet a need of nursing and the organization.** Both Kramer and Van Slyck met specific needs. Kramer, through her collaboration with the HSRA, conducted research, published their outcomes, and presented their work across the United States. Van Slyck and her company, Van Slyck and Associates, consulted, created tools, published, and presented throughout the United States.

In summary, when collaboration and wisdom sharing are recognized and used, untold potential is unleashed, and the possibilities that emerge contribute significantly to the profession and science of nursing.

RECOGNIZING AND CELEBRATING

Is there a role for recognizing and celebrating transitions beyond retirement parties and plaques commemorating one's work years and professional accomplishments? If so, what is the role of recognition and celebration with regard to transferring knowledge and formally marking one's passage while securing connections for the future? For those of us from the baby boomer generation, how do we choose and create the type of celebrations that are meaningful to us as we transition? What is the link between these celebrations and relationships that lead to accomplishing meaningful future goals?

Merriam-Webster (n.d.) defines *celebrate* as "to mark with an appropriate practice, rite, or ceremony" and defines *recognition* as "special notice or attention." These definitions make us ask, "What is the appropriate practice, rite, or ceremony, and how do we take special notice of this transition?"

As a result of Kramer's leadership, seminal publications, and perseverance during her professional work that spanned more than 5 decades, in 2012 she was awarded the Anthony J. Jannetti "Tony" Award for Extraordinary Contributions to Healthcare by the Academy of Medical-Surgical Nurses (AMSN). Kramer agreed that honors and awards are important, and although she received many, her most significant honor was this "lifetime achievement award" because it represented the practice and views of medical-surgical nurses who work in hundreds of hospitals all over the United States. Nurses in this specialty have always kept Kramer grounded in the reality of professional nursing practice at the bedside, which she values.

"It is literally true that you can succeed best and quickest by helping others to succeed."
—Napoleon Hill

At the 2012 AMSN national conference, Kramer had the opportunity to address the 1,000-plus nurses in attendance. These nurses, who are likely the best, brightest, and most professionally involved nurses in their field, represented hundreds of hospitals, and Kramer was able to meet with them, interview them, and discuss relevant issues these nurses were grappling with in their practice. The dialogues continued over email and span the years as nurses continue to pose questions to Kramer and scenarios that have not yet been addressed to their satisfaction within their employment organizations or professional organizations. Kramer continues to see the world through their eyes and experiences, which continues to inform the research questions and study designs that the nurse scientists of HSRA then address.

When we mentioned the topic of recognition and celebration as a strategy to support transitioning to Van Slyck, she quietly sat for a few minutes and then stated, "I need to get out of the way. I am living in the in-between. I am recognizing, celebrating, and appreciating what has been, and I am letting go of what was so that I can create space for the 'not yets.'" Regarding her contributions to the science of nursing and the creation of a thriving business, Van Slyck remarked that if the work is important, it will live on even after Van Slyck is no longer involved. She too received a lifetime achievement award in 2009, which was bestowed upon her by the American Organization of Nurse Executives.

How did Van Slyck celebrate her personal endings related to her first passion—assisting nurse leaders in patient classification and celebrating what she had yet to offer? Her own professional and financial success allowed her to refocus her energy on birthing a new passion. She shifted her contributions from determining the care needs of patients to providing the actual equipment, beds, and supplies needed to provide that care. She used her business-savvy and her resourceful, persuasive, passionate, and compassionate traits to secure the delivery of more than $1 million of medical supplies to five hospitals in Sri Lanka.

Van Slyck's maxim in life has served her well: "If you can't change it, accept it; and if you can't accept it, change it." She also believes that "the journey to success is an evolution, and every success brings a new circumstance. It's OK to be afraid. Just keep moving forward."

PRINCIPLES OF RECOGNIZING AND CELEBRATING

The following principles emerged from the Kramer and Van Slyck interviews:

- **Receiving personally meaningful awards.** Both Kramer and Van Slyck received lifetime achievement awards that recognized and publicized their contributions to their respective areas of practice and provided the opportunity for others to remain connected with them as they each continued expanding their work and contributing to the art and science of nursing practice.

- **Handing off to others.** As Kramer's collaborators continued researching, publishing, and presenting as members of the HSRA consortium, she was in a position to hand off the role of president and leadership to others within the consortium so that the work would continue and she could pursue other passions. Van Slyck also handled her handoff in a unique way. She sold her company to a larger entity that would pursue patient acuity, which allowed Van Slyck to explore a newly emerging passion.

Even though public recognition and celebration may have a fleeting impact for those of us who are witnesses, the possibilities of what can be are only realized following transitions by the ones who are recognized and celebrated. As seen in both exemplars, valued outcomes result for both leaders, the legacy of practice environment research in Kramer's case and the space to contribute and create in new ways in Van Slyck's case.

PERSONAL APPLICATION

The following questions are designed to help you reflect on the knowledge and wisdom you have gained over your career and to facilitate the successful transfer of this knowledge and wisdom to those nurse leaders who, like you, have devoted their life's work to their patients and to the nursing profession.

1. Storytelling is an effective strategy to convey organizational culture in a compelling and memorable manner.

   - What stories do you want to tell? Think of those experiences that were very impactful on your career—those ah-ha moments, now that you reflect on them, that were transformational to you early in your career.

   - How can you provide the story that captures your insights and learnings to share with others?

2. The support and guidance of a trusted mentor can contribute to a valuable leadership experience.

   - Whom do you want to mentor?

   - How can you support the growth and development of someone you know who has great potential?

   - If you are currently mentoring someone, what insights did you obtain from this chapter that could enhance that mentoring relationship?

3. Questions can lead to intriguing new possibilities.

   - What reminders can you put in place to increase the application of powerful questions (start using questions that begin with "what" and "how")?

   - How can you use powerful questions more often?

4. Continuous career planning and skill enhancement are necessities in today's ever-changing healthcare environment. Knowing your strengths, goals, and aspirations is key to creating, managing, and evaluating your career options.

   - How can you share career options and insights and assist individuals early in their career?

   - As you explore career options, whom can you connect with to gain insights about career options?

5. Collaboration is an essential component of creating meaningful relationships, and it is conducive to sharing our wisdom.

   - What is your passion and vision in your chosen area of specialization?

   - Who are the like-minded professional colleagues who can nurture, contribute to, and sustain the work in your specialty?

   - How can you and your colleagues' collaborative efforts contribute to the science and/or discipline of nursing?

6. Recognition and celebration can be both noble and energizing and can serve as meaningful markers along one's nursing career.

   - What is an award that you would like to strive for that would serve as significant recognition of your contributions to our profession?

   - As you think about your own career handoff, what would bring you joy and cause for celebration?

LOOKING FORWARD

It is through deliberate efforts and actions of both seasoned, wise, experienced leaders and early-career, emerging leaders that connections are made, and the two groups can co-create the future by cultivating key relationships and intentionally capturing and nurturing the wisdom of the generations. The six strategies that were discussed serve as guides that can lead to building effective, trusting relationships, which is the bedrock upon which we can advance both the art and science of nursing.

"By learning you will teach, by teaching you will learn."
–Latin proverb

7
LIFELONG LEARNING AND GIVING

OLIVIA QUIST
ADRIENNE LYONS, MSN, RN

CHAPTER OBJECTIVES

Identify selected sources of online adult education.

Describe considerations of the mature adult in obtaining an advanced academic degree.

Identify various venues where healthcare practitioners acting in a volunteer capacity can positively impact both local and global initiatives.

This old Latin proverb "By learning you will teach, by teaching you will learn" sets the stage for this chapter, which is dedicated to lifelong learning, reciprocal teaching, and giving back. In this chapter we present lessons for the next generation of leaders, who will maximize their personal and professional potential by internalizing a commitment to learning at every stage of life. We believe that by developing an appreciation for ongoing education and actively pursuing enrichment activities, we have provided a model for both aging well and remaining relevant in this fast-paced and evolving healthcare environment. In planning for and developing the next generation of leaders, we hope to lead by exemplifying the benefits and delight of ongoing education and giving back.

This chapter is written from two distinct perspectives. It expresses the thoughts and experiences of two women with a combined 143 years of living and thriving in two distinct fields. Both are exemplars of lifelong learning. In her 60s, Adrienne Lyons chose to enter a formal, structured academic program to pursue a doctor of nursing practice degree. Olivia Quist, a successful real estate businesswoman of 80 years, is still practicing and productive in her field, and she continues to master numerous new skills.

These are the questions we asked ourselves and have done our best to answer in the chapter:

- What lessons have we learned on our journeys that may be of interest and relevance to the upcoming group of practitioners?

- What lessons must be scrapped, revised, or reinvented to become relevant and useful to the next group?

- What have we learned about staying involved, productive, and committed to our own personal development?

- How are we managing to stay in the game and age with passion and purpose?

The growth in the number and proportion of older adults is unprecedented in the history of the United States. Two factors—longer life spans and aging baby boomers—will combine to double the population of Americans aged 65 years or older during the next 25 years, bringing the total to about 72 million. According to the Centers for Disease Control and Prevention (2013), by 2030, older adults will account for roughly 20% of the U.S. population.

According to the MacArthur Foundation Research Network on an Aging Society (2008), in the past century, the life expectancy of individuals in the United States has risen from 47 to 77 years as seniors avail themselves of healthcare that has made significant technological advances. The same report notes that by the middle of the 2020 decade, it is predicted that there will be more people in their 60s than people under age 15. This fast-growing and generally healthy generation may be redefining aging with a vital lifestyle. With advances in healthcare, many are able to live with good health well into their 80s and 90s. This phenomenon impacts the nursing workforce also. There will be more people needing healthcare, especially with the baby boomers who value a healthy aging process and seek care to promote health and avoid illness.

An extended life expectancy provides for additional time to pass along wisdom gained through the years. The nursing community may be enriched by this. Front-line nursing staff who are staying in the profession longer and healthier can continue to mentor and encourage the novice nurse. It is also true for nurse managers as they focus on developing themselves and their staffs to perfect their practice and produce better outcomes. Nurse leaders and executives have a unique opportunity to impact the larger healthcare community by leveraging their knowledge, experience, and credibility to improve care delivery. Many nurse leaders in our community actively dialogue with their legislators to advocate for various healthcare and professional issues. Not only are these nurse leaders providing a vital perspective, but they are also setting an example for those nurses who will follow them to actively participate in the process of healthcare regulation and funding. Nurse leaders should consider engaging younger nurses to accompany them to meeting with decision-makers. Of course, to assume the role of expert, leaders must continually refresh their knowledge and actively pursue learning opportunities both within and outside of their field.

○---▶

"Anyone can get old. All you have to do is live long enough."
—Groucho Marx

LEADING BY EXAMPLE

There is a nurse executive in my community whom I greatly admire for many reasons. He established a quarterly journal club and actively participates in leading discussions on current topics. Several years ago, he realized that learning was beginning to occur in electronic formats, especially with the younger, technically adept nurses, so he converted his traditional club into an online club. Staff members were impressed that he was willing to learn this new skill to meet their needs. By the way, he has also learned to play the guitar and has become a certified scuba diver. He humorously discusses his struggles with new skill acquisition in his monthly blog to the staff, titled "Old Dogs." What a great example he is setting.

—Adrienne Lyons, MSN, RN

LIFELONG LEARNING

With aging comes the probability of retirement from the traditional workforce. Unemployment may be frightening to many, because of both financial and self-esteem considerations. We have often worked to live: to establish a lifestyle that allows us to become property owners, raise and educate children, and create savings. A professional life and parenting bring a lot of energy and purpose to life. With aging and the diminishing influence of these motivating factors, it might become necessary to find alternative sources of energy and purpose. When the traditional work life concludes, many individuals feel the need to continue a productive life and develop a lifestyle that holds pleasure and meaning. It might not be enough to transition to a life of leisure. Without a career, seniors are liberated to pursue their own passions and interests. Part of the wisdom that we would like to hand off is the importance of planning for what might be one-third of your life by learning new skills and redirecting well-honed skills—in other words, continuing to learn your entire life.

The exciting thing about lifelong learning is that it never stops! During your working career, your focus is naturally on learning more about your profession. But as we achieve competency in our profession and perhaps have a little more time, there is often a desire to pursue other areas of knowledge. Perhaps you have always wanted to play a musical instrument or learn to dance the tango. Maybe you would like to understand the U.S. Constitution or travel to Machu Picchu. Some people want to trace their family history and visit the homeland of their ancestors. Others want to learn to paint, draw, quilt, arrange flowers, or cook gourmet meals. Education in other disciplines, different from our careers, creates a balance in our life. It opens up new perspectives, taps into neglected parts of our abilities, enriches our life, and might even prevent dementia. In his book *Master Class: Living Longer, Stronger, and Happier*, Peter Spiers (2012) identifies four dimensions that contribute to successful aging: socializing, moving, thinking, and creating. "Why are these four dimensions so important? They're important because, together, they are the key elements of a holistic way of life that will bring you happiness, optimism, and physical and cognitive health."

AGING SUCCESSFULLY

One of the authors, Olivia Quist, leads a life full of healthy physical and intellectual activities that contribute to each of the four dimensions that Spiers (2012) identifies as successful aging. A look into a week of 82-year-old Quist's life reveals daily walks—usually at least 1.5 miles—and participation in weekly yoga, aqua, and senior fitness classes (moving). She enjoys practicing her culinary skills and is writing a history of her pioneer ranching family (creating). She is usually involved in academic courses, such as classical music and current film history, accessed either locally or online (thinking). Her love of books draws her to several book clubs and discussion groups (thinking and socializing). She meditates daily. She remains active in her real estate profession and holds open houses, shows properties, and writes contracts for buying homes, but she is handing off her business of 35 years to her daughter (moving, thinking, and creating and handing off to the younger generation). Even with all these pursuits, Quist still has time for family and community activities.

In the following sections we share with you ideas to facilitate your quest for lifelong learning. You can find opportunities for learning in formal classes, book clubs, travel, physical activity, and advanced degrees. We encourage you to challenge yourself to try some activities that you have not done before.

EDUCATIONAL COURSES

Massive open online courses (MOOCs) are a fascinating resource for learning on the Internet, and many of these MOOCs are free of charge. Offered by a wealth of universities and taught by highly respected professors, the number of courses offered has exploded in recent years. Learning happens in several ways: the professor's knowledge, your personal exploration of the subject, and the online interaction with other students taking the class. The views and comments of fellow students from different age groups, nationalities, and levels of expertise in the subject enrich the learning experience. These courses are truly intergenerational experiences because of the questions and insights that students of all ages post.

An Internet search will result in a long list of institutions offering courses. You can also search for a specific university, such as Yale University or a favorite university in your home state or abroad. Table 7.1 includes the starting points we recommend. The websites for these organizations include options for you to sign up for newsletters or emails that will notify you when classes that match your interests are being offered.

TABLE 7.1: OPPORTUNITIES FOR ONLINE EDUCATION

Organization	Focus	Website
Udacity	Vocational courses for professionals in information technology (IT)	https://www.udacity.com
Class Central	Online courses from top universities, such as Stanford University, Massachusetts Institute of Technology (MIT), and Harvard University	https://www.class-central.com
edX	Online university-level courses in a wide range of disciplines	https://www.edx.org
Coursera	Online courses partnering with top universities and organizations	https://www.coursera.org

Another great source for university-level classes is The Great Courses (http://www.thegreatcourses.com). The classes can be purchased or checked out from the library in CD, DVD, and audio or video download format. Course subjects include science, history, professional training, mathematics, economics, fine arts, music, and more. You can listen to CDs in your car or gather a group to watch video lectures and then discuss them.

TRAVEL

Travel and learning are a great combination whether you are traveling solo or in an organized group. Road Scholar (http://www.roadscholar. org), formerly Elderhostel, is a nonprofit organization that offers more than 5,500 educational tours in all 50 U.S. states and 150 countries. You can choose from cultural tours, study cruises, or walking and biking tours. Many universities, such as Cornell Adult Vacations and St. John's College, offer classes on campus in the off-season. Shaw Guides (http://www.shawguides.com) provides information about travel to study culinary arts, writer's workshops, language classes, tennis, golf, and extreme sports. Or you can plan your own itinerary to wherever your interests lead you.

○---▶
"Not all who wander are lost."
–J.R.R. Tolkien

TRAVELING WITH INTENTION

One family who went to Sweden to research their family roots did advance planning. They contacted the Swedish government, which has a department to research emigrants using the Lutheran Church records. The travelers then located members from both maternal and fraternal families and wrote to them about the upcoming visit. They also watched the 1971 Swedish film *The Emigrants,* which traces a family moving from Sweden to Minnesota in the 19th century, as this family's ancestors had. They read a book on Swedish history and art. This advance planning made the trip much more interesting than it might otherwise have been because they were able to visit relatives in their homes and find the grave sites of ancestors who had died in the 1700s. The family knew which museums they wanted to visit and the route their trip would take. The trip helped them imagine what life had been like for their ancestors and why and how they emigrated to North America. They were able to fill in many spaces on the family tree, which they can hand down to future generations. Returning home, the husband wrote a book about his family, which included the history gathered on their travels.

PHYSICAL ACTIVITY

Throughout our lives we are encouraged to get physical exercise. Unfortunately, many people who age, even if they were formerly active, give up on exercise. Perhaps they have a physical limitation or they lose interest in a sport because their skill level is diminished. Almost without exception, there is some form of exercise appropriate for all. For example, yoga can be modified to be done by someone who is seated in a chair. Janet Rae Humphrey, a teacher in Arizona, won a yoga contest with her video of 90-year-olds in her class (http://www.YogaForStability.com). *Time* magazine published a feature article titled "Why Tai Chi Is the Perfect Exercise" (July 31, 2002). Almost everyone can do some light weight lifting, which many experts believe is as important as aerobic training. Walking is a simple exercise and requires no formal affiliation or training. It is fun to try physical activities you have never done before, thereby stimulating brain function as well as muscles. What is the best exercise? Any exercise that you will do regularly.

BOOK CLUBS

Discussing books can create an atmosphere of sharing of experience and knowledge that can pass both ways between older and younger members. It is estimated that more than 5 million people are in reading groups (Heller, 2011). They are formed by young and old, men and women. In large part their popularity is due to the sociability component that occurs within the group. Book clubs can increase your knowledge and provide teaching moments; they can include inter-generational members.

If you decide to have a group that meets in person, you need to choose a meeting place, decide on a convenient time, and invite members. Books can be chosen by the leader or the whole group. For good discussions it is optimal to limit the group to between 12 and 15 members (larger groups might require longer meetings for members to participate fully). Also, it is helpful to have a facilitator for the discussion.

Online book clubs are also effective. Advantages include flexible times to participate and no restriction on the number of members. (It is hard to provide electronic wine and cheese, however.) You can post discussion questions to a group's Facebook page or other social media sites and hold a "Go to Meeting" final discussion. As with groups that meet face-to-face, online book clubs need to choose the books and have a leader who keeps the group going.

For suggestions of books to read and for book reviews, consider checking out the American Library Association (http://www.booklistonline.com), Goodreads (http://www.goodreads.com/list), and Modern Library (http://www.modernlibrary.com/top-100).

ADVANCED DEGREES

A more formal approach to lifelong learning may appeal to some. As I was contemplating returning to academia to pursue a doctor of nursing practice degree, my primary concern was, "When are you too old to attempt an advanced degree?" I finally concluded, "If you are motivated and curious—never!" However, before embarking on returning to school, I recommend that you fully explore your

"Live as if you were to die tomorrow. Learn as if you were to live forever."
—Mahatma Gandhi

motivation. Are you in your 50s with a desire to further your present career? Are you in your 60s and want to advance your knowledge base? Are you looking to completely retool yourself and master new knowledge and skills?

However, older adults must consider several variables in addition to having a strong desire to enter a degree program. In particular, the time required to be successful in coursework cannot be underestimated. Also, the considerable cost of the program should be fully explored prior to committing. There might be fewer scholarships and financial aid awarded to older students, and navigating the options may be challenging. An older applicant may have concerns related to a favorable decision from the selection committee. Is age a barrier? Will subtle age discrimination be a factor? Surely the older applicant has fewer years of productivity and potential contributions to the field as well as fewer years to conduct research and publish. If the applicant's goal is to be on the faculty, attaining tenure may be unlikely. All of these issues may inform the decision for program admission.

With those cautions in mind, applicants would be wise to explore their own capacity for resilience and flexibility. Older individuals might have many years of success in the work environment, which is comfortable and safe. They might have been recognized and respected for their expertise. Will they be able to let go of those former roles and thrive in the role of novice student? Although older individuals may have enthusiasm for such a bold change, do they have the emotional maturity and flexibility to redefine themselves? Another very practical consideration is whether the older adult possesses adequate technological skills to navigate the new educational environment. Joyce, a doctoral student in her late 50s, revealed, "I have always had an administrative assistant who prepared my documents, PowerPoints, and presentations. In the student role I knew that support would not be available. I had to enroll in introductory computer classes to learn the basics before I could take my first doctoral course." The literature supports that healthy adults are capable of learning well into their 70s and 80s (Crawford, 2004). So, while assimilating new knowledge might require more concentration and time commitment, seniors are capable of demonstrating the ability.

We have discussed the implications for formal learning on the aging adult, but there are also implications for the academic community in terms of capturing this rapidly expanding demographic. The American Council on Education (2015) recently published its first report on older adults and higher education. The report noted that the primary motivators of "elderlearners" are intellectual stimulation, skills enhancement, and the opportunity to socialize. Programming and class design are beginning to acknowledge the older student. Distance learning and online courses are numerous and negate barriers such as mobility and transportation access, yet that format does not address the older student's desire to be a part of a community. Support services may not be designed to meet the needs of older learners. Blended or hybrid courses incorporating onsite and online learning opportunities might appeal to those who seek a personal touch but want convenience and flexibility for class time and location.

In addition, some older students perceive a negative attitude from instructors. Mary entered a doctoral program at age 55 and described an attitude of impatience by faculty. She was told, "You are well experienced in your field and should not have to ask so many questions and constantly seek clarity." The broad diversity of older adults in terms of experience, interests, and talents challenges both formal and informal educators to tailor programs to engage this group. The additional issues of race, ethnicity, and income have not been well studied but should be considered.

EXPERIENCE SHOULD COUNT

As I entered a doctor of nursing practice program, I was confident that I was a self-directed learner who brought an extensive background in nursing leadership and clinical practice. I was surprised to learn that the program did not acknowledge my 25+ years of acquired expertise and required that I complete multiple clinical practicums. However, I chose to proceed and actually looked forward to the experiences that I would encounter in multiple settings. However, more learner control in the selection of practicums would have been welcome. Ideally, the selection committee would have been more open to acknowledgment of my many years of healthcare experience as it pertained to my course of study.

—Adrienne Lyons, MSN, RN

GIVING BACK AS A VOLUNTEER

Learning and giving back are complementary activities. Many older people are no longer in the traditional workforce but still have a strong desire to be useful and productive. Many seniors have a clear sense of their past, which they view with pride, but they might now feel the need to define a different future. There are numerous volunteer opportunities for the aging to fulfill their sense of commitment to a community, project, or cause. The role of the volunteer may replace what was lost in retirement as the concept of aging is transforming from one of poor health and frailty to one of an active, talented, and giving asset. Volunteering provides a connection and common purpose and may prevent the isolation of aging. According to the Corporation for National and Community Service (2013), 28% of baby boomers participated in volunteer activities in 2013, with 280 million hours of valuable and needed services provided.

Volunteering usually is not a response to external pressure, but rather is driven from an inner source. Typically, there is no ulterior motive. This drive may be especially evident in older nurses who have spent their careers nurturing others and now seek opportunities to continue that inner purpose that does not diminish simply because one has retired. Skilled executives and professionals might be looking for important and creative roles as mentors and volunteers for nonprofits, which might benefit from the knowledge of successful seniors who do not want to operate at the feverish pace of a competitive formal work environment.

Volunteerism is rich with opportunities to expand horizons, bolster personal growth, provide fun, increase one's circle of acquaintances, and provide self-satisfaction. If you are interested in exploring volunteer opportunities, Tables 7.2 and 7.3 provide descriptions of several worthy organizations and their contact information.

TABLE 7.2: RESOURCES FOR SENIOR VOLUNTEERS

Organization	Focus	Website
Seniors Corps	Connects seniors with organizations as mentors, coaches, or companions to people in need, or as experts in community projects and organizations	www.nationalservice.gov/programs/senior-corps
International Service Corps	Taps volunteers to work in the areas of trade, enterprise, information communication technologies, financial services, tourism, and the public sector	www.iesc.org

Retired Seniors Volunteer Program	Provides opportunities for caring for children, teaching conversational English, assisting with building repair and painting, and planting and maintaining community gardens	www.globalvolunteers.org
Habitat for Humanity and Jimmy Carter Work Project	Offers opportunities to build stable housing locally and abroad	www.habitat.org
Experience Corps	Sets up older adults as student literacy tutors	www.aarp.org/ experience-corps

TABLE 7.3: RESOURCES FOR REGISTERED NURSE VOLUNTEERS

Organization	Focus	Website
Red Cross	Public health local and abroad, disaster relief	www.redcross.org
American Nurses Association	Emergency response	www.nursingworld.org
Nurse Without Borders	Promote and provide medical care	www.nursewithoutborders.org
Doctors Without Borders	Basic healthcare and disaster relief	www.doctorswithoutborders.org

Within nursing, volunteer opportunities exist that serve to both foster professional development and contribute to the common good. Even as a young nurse, all of my mentors encouraged me (Adrienne) to become active in professional organizations. Through the years I did attend meetings and events, but usually as an observer. It was only when I realized that I had the skill to assume leadership roles that I truly understood what my more senior and experienced nurse mentors expected of me. My unabashed love of food led me to become involved with my local food pantry and distribution center. Helping a client choose the more healthy options available and participating in nutrition classes have met a need in me to be involved with feeding people, something in which I take great pleasure even in my own kitchen.

PERSONAL APPLICATION

The following questions are designed to help you reflect on the knowledge and wisdom you have gained over your career and to facilitate the successful transfer of this knowledge and wisdom to those nurse leaders who, like you, have devoted their life's work to their patients and to the nursing profession.

1. Nurses have an important opportunity on their professional journey to learn from older coworkers, especially those who serve in a formal mentorship role.

   - Do you have a mentor who freely offers an experienced perspective?
   - If not, do you have an opportunity to identify a mentor and form a mutually beneficial relationship?
   - What is the best advice you ever received from a mentor?

2. Older professionals can share much wisdom with their younger coworkers.

   - What is the best advice you have passed along?
   - Have you supported a workplace culture of respect for inquiry?
   - Do you promote constant examination of rituals and sacred cows in the workplace to effect positive change?
   - Are you teaching your younger colleagues the joy of mentorship—and if so, how?

3. No matter the stage of your professional life, a practice of lifelong learning will enable you to remain relevant.

- What opportunities do you have in your life to travel and appreciate diversity?
- What activities are available to keep you current?

4. Giving back to your community may be a valuable use of your time, talent, and energy.

- What value do you see in volunteering your time and talent?
- What are some causes or organizations that are of interest to you? Is there an opportunity to assume a leadership position or influence the work to achieve the best outcomes for those you serve, or do you prefer working in support roles?

5. Passion and purpose must be fueled, and lifelong learning plays a key part in keeping your passion and purpose fresh and exciting.

- Do you jump in and try new experiences? Why or why not?
- Do you read or join discussion groups either in person or online?
- How do such activities fuel your desires and goals?

LOOKING FORWARD

We hope the information and experiences in this chapter have been helpful. Our goal is to provide readers with the benefits and delights of pursuing challenging educational opportunities and leading an active lifestyle to nurture oneself and one's profession, create a satisfying retirement, and perhaps fulfill lifelong dreams. Learning can give purpose, meaning, and joy to our lives, even in later years. Sharing our skills and knowledge can extend beyond personal fulfillment and dreams to include a contribution to the health of society. We have both faced challenges in keeping current in our respective vocations. All of the effort has involved advanced education of one kind or another, with the overarching goal of handing off hard-won wisdom to the next generation. We have discussed with each other the many activities within our scopes. In the end, we determined that all of our advice for the next generation emanates from the simple concept of committing to a life guided by a constant spirit of inquiry and personal improvement. To the next generation, we encourage you to:

- Question everything.
- Set goals and execute strategies that are based on strong evidence.
- Recognize that the status quo is not sacred. Research a better method.
- Lead to effect positive change.
- Build personal credibility by passionately advocating for change.
- Consider that working in the spotlight is not always the best approach.
- Continuously search for and collaborate with mentors.

We also suggest:

- Jumping in
- Participating
- Volunteering
- Reading and writing

At the Nobel Museum in Stockholm, Sweden, laureates from many disciplines are commemorated for their inspiration, role modeling, and the value of passing on wisdom. The plaque at the entry states simply this:

Legacy
Leave your world a better place than it was.

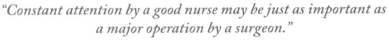

*"Constant attention by a good nurse may be just as important as
a major operation by a surgeon."*

–Dag Hammarskjold

8

LEAVING NURSING BETTER THAN YOU FOUND IT

GREGORY CROW, EDD, RN

CHAPTER OBJECTIVES

Analyze how paradigms affect our perspective on nursing.

Analyze the impact of bullying in academic and practice environments.

Analyze the accountability that deans and administrators in practice environments have in combating bullying.

Define pay it forward (PIF).

Apply the PIF model to nurse educators, point-of-care nurses, and nurse administrators.

Analyze how components of being future-focused can create nursing's preferred future.

Before beginning this chapter, I would like to emphasize the importance of the content conveyed in the preceding chapters. Every nurse must learn and internalize this knowledge and insight because it provides a wonderful and timely foundation for nursing's future. Each of us has the obligation to welcome the next generation of nurses into our profession. It is our responsibility to help our new colleagues develop the necessary knowledge, skills, and abilities that will create a strong foundation on which to build their practice and to improve nursing overall. This chapter discusses the obligation that we all have as nurses to leave our profession in better condition than we found it.

The impetus for this chapter came to me while I was doing data analysis for a qualitative research study that three colleagues and I are conducting on the meaning of being a nurse in an intensive care unit in Ha Noi, Vietnam. A prominent theme noted by each of the researchers was the positive relationship between the senior/experienced nurse and the early-career nurse. The early-career nurses acknowledged how much they appreciated the thoughtful guidance they received from the senior/ experienced nurses and their head nurse. Because they reported similar positive relationships during their nursing school clinical experiences, they anticipated that this support would continue as they entered the profession.

Throughout the nearly 10 years that I have been the director of the Vietnam Nurse Project (VNP) at the University of San Francisco, School of Nursing and Health Professions, San Francisco, California, I have noticed a trustful and respectful relationship among nurses in Vietnam. This is quite the opposite of the "eating our young" attitude that is sometimes prevalent in U.S. nursing culture. When I shared the "eating our young" concept with my Vietnamese nurse colleagues, they were shocked and could not see any advantage or benefit to this type of behavior. Although I am not naive enough to believe that this type of behavior doesn't exist in Vietnam, I can say with great confidence that it is not part of their practice when welcoming new nurses into the profession. I believe that nurses in the United States could learn a great deal from their Vietnamese colleagues about caring and compassion among all generations of nurses. Cooperation is so integrated into the Vietnamese nursing culture that every VNP volunteer who has traveled to Vietnam with us has noticed and commented about it.

NURSE IDENTITY

Walker et al. (2014) note that one's professional identity can guide or narrow an individual's satisfaction with his or her role. Additionally, they note that there are actually two identities we develop as a nurse: our individual identity and our collective identity as a professional group.

I believe that a modicum of positive tension between the individual identity and the collective identity of every nurse is necessary. That positive tension is the space where nurses, no matter their current role, emerge from the existing paradigm of nursing and transition to a new paradigm that is more likely to meet the varied, complex, and ever-changing needs of the public we serve. It also provides new roles for nurses, such as clinical nurse leader and the doctorate in nursing practice. These roles were unthinkable only a few years ago. Barker (1992) calls these individuals "paradigm pioneers." Florence Nightingale is the ultimate role model.

Nightingale (1969) said it best when describing the nursing paradigm that she inherited: "The accepted idea of the time was that nothing but a disappointment in love, or incapacity in other things, was required to turn a woman into a good nurse" (p. xii). Nightingale's time was many generations before the women's movement, and the thinking at that time was that nursing could only attract people with lower social status.

Lavinia Dock and Isabel Stewart (1931) described paradigm
pioneers as:

> The movement which revolutionized modern nursing has car-
> ried us forward by its great impetus to the present time. The
> question now is, whether we shall slip back with one of those
> ebb tides of reaction so familiar in history when the momen-
> tum of a great movement slackens, and the pioneers of that
> movement begin to give way to a new generation (p. 347).

To put that statement into contemporary terms, each generation of
nurses has to expand the nursing paradigm that the last generation constructed on their behalf, even if that paradigm feels comfortable. In fact,
if it is comfortable, you should plan your escape sooner than later. If you
stay where the last generation of nurses left nursing, Barker (1992) tells
us you suffer from the terminal disease
of "paradigm paralysis." *Paradigm pa-*
ralysis prevents individuals from having
a wider worldview, restricts possibilities, and can damage any profession.
Nothing could be worse for a professional or profession than to find comfort in this terminal disease.

*"You never change things by
fighting the existing reality. To
change something, build a new
model that makes the existing
model obsolete."*
–R. Buckminster Fuller

Paradigm pioneers see what others cannot (Barker, 1992) and often are
those nurses who tinker around the edges of nursing practice domains.
As mentioned earlier, having paradigm pioneers who saw practice
boundaries as opportunities resulted in the creation of the certified registered nurse anesthetist role, one of the first advanced practice roles for
nurses. Being a paradigm pioneer is not the easiest job in the world; just
ask anyone who has introduced a new idea to colleagues and managers
and received a rejection even before the idea could be adequately ex-

plained or explored. We need to say, "Tell me more," rather than, "That idea won't work."

Without the vision and work of paradigm pioneers, we would not have baccalaureate, master's, or doctoral programs in nursing, nor would we have a nurse practice act independent of medicine. Without paradigm pioneers, our nursing schools would still be under the direct control of physicians whose primary interest was often to produce a good assistant for themselves—not to develop nursing as an independent profession. We would not have advanced practice nurses such as clinical nurse specialists, nurse practitioners, and certified registered nurse anesthetists. Paradigm pioneers in these areas chartered a course that benefited all nurses, just as clinical nurse leaders and doctorate in nursing practice nurses are doing now.

THE NEW NURSE

In my nearly 40 years of nursing experience as student nurse, staff nurse, nurse recruiter, supervisor, professor, administrator, consultant, and director of a nongovernmental organization in a foreign country, many of the undergraduate and master's entry students have a very narrow view of what nurses do. For many potential students, the concept of what a nurse does is often formed by popular literature, film, and television— not the best sources for choosing a career. It is important for faculty to understand that an individual's identity as a nurse begins long before enrolling in nursing school.

Although students attend nursing school for many reasons, frequent motives are explained by statements such as, "I like to help people"; "My mother or father is/was a nurse"; and "I was a patient, and the nurses really helped me." Unfortunately, there are also those students who say, "My parents made me go to nursing school." Faculty has the obligation to clearly understand students' motivations for entering nursing school and to assist them in clarifying the general role of the nurse. Moreover, nursing schools are obligated to help potential students better understand their motivation and inspiration for entering nursing and to help them determine if nursing is a good fit for them. Not everyone can or should be a nurse.

In August 1974, during my last days as a corpsman in the United States Air Force, Major Doris Woodward, RN, said to me, "Now that you have decided to become a nurse, treat it well." Major Woodward's words have stuck with me to this day and have guided my stitched-together career in a profession that I love, and a profession that has provided me with unlimited possibilities and opportunities for learning and practice. The best decision I ever made was to become a nurse.

After graduating nursing school in 1977, I took a practice opportunity at a 250-bed community hospital in northern California, knowing that I had been thrust into a new role as a paradigm pioneer. I was one of 12 new graduates hired directly into the intensive care units (ICU) at that hospital. In many places in the United States, taking a new graduate into the ICU was thought of as crazy. New graduates at the time were often told that there was only one path to get to the ICU (as a nurse), and that was through 3 to 5 years in medical-surgical nursing. I remember asking why I needed to spend those years in medical-surgical nursing when critical-care nursing was my goal. The answer was always the same, "Because that was the way I got to practice in the ICU." That statement is an excellent example of paradigm paralysis.

The attitude that new graduate nurses were not capable of functioning in ICUs was a core belief of many nurses and physicians. Those naysayers were surprised as they met a force named Jackie Jewell, RN, who was head nurse of the acute cardiac care unit where I was hired as a new graduate nurse. She believed that with careful guidance and nurturing, new graduates would, in time, perform as well as experienced nurses. Jackie was right, and she made sure that each of us knew she would support us in an environment that did not think we should be there. Most important, she would help us win over the existing staff. Jackie also informed us that we were paving the way for the next class of new graduates in critical care, and if we did well, they would do well.

What this important paradigm pioneer role taught me was that uncertainty is survivable; change is not a four-letter word in disguise; and, most important, having a great leader makes all the difference in the world. I learned these incredible lessons in my first year as a registered nurse. That experience left an indelible imprint on me and has guided me throughout my career.

THE HIRING PROCESS

In preparing this chapter, I also had to delve into the darker side of our nursing culture. It is the aspect of nursing that is harmful to students, practicing nurses (academia and clinical practice), and the nursing profession as a whole. It is important for each of us to know when we are helping the profession to grow and develop rather than harming it through incompetence as a practicing nurse or a faculty member. Although I believe that we must give people the opportunity to improve, we must also be realistic and face the facts that uncivil behavior in universities and clinical practice environments does a great deal of damage to the individual nurse and to nursing as a whole.

When academic and healthcare organizations hire faculty and staff, they generally pay much more attention to the candidate's technical and theoretical knowledge than to his or her interpersonal skills. Consider that I can teach almost anyone to construct an inspiring course and how to masterfully deliver the subject in a way that enhances the ability of the students to learn, internalize the materials, and apply their knowledge in real clinical situations. Moreover, I can teach almost anyone to start an IV, insert a nasogastric tube, interpret lab results, mix and calculate medications, and master the process of the head-to-toe physical assessment. It is, however, incredibly difficult to teach an adult to be a nice person. And if the people themselves cannot recognize that their behavior is harming other nurses, potentially harming patients, or harming nursing at large, then the professionals who they report to must take action and help them to see how their behavior negatively affects teamwork and unit cohesion, both of which are vital to good patient outcomes. Nurse leaders must then provide the disruptive nurse with support on how to change and improve. Moreover, if the nurse does not change within a specified time frame, the nurse should be separated from the organization.

In most cases, chronic disruptive behavior is a basic math issue: It costs far less to refresh or introduce new skills than to address the lack of interpersonal skills, of which "horizontal violence" and "bullying" are the prime examples. Moreover, bullying has a significant financial impact on organizations. Gerardia and Connell (2007) and Pendry (2007), as cited by Becher and Visovsky (2012), provide financial estimates of the impact of bullying. They note that bullying can cost an organization between $30,000 and $100,000 per year for each individual who is bullied. The costs are associated with absenteeism, treatment for depression and anxiety, decreased work performance, and early-career nurse and experienced-nurse turnover. It is estimated that replacing one specialty nurse may exceed $145,000 when taking into account recruiting, training, and orientation. At a time when every penny counts toward organizational success, it amazes me that we are willing to spend money on people who have clearly demonstrated they are not willing to change.

EATING OUR YOUNG: THE BULLY IN ACTION

Before discussing the bully in action, I would like to remind the reader that "...alleviation of suffering..." (ANA, 2015b) is a very important characteristic that defines nursing. The literature is replete with research and narrative articles regarding how bullying leads to suffering. As mentioned earlier, the costs can be as high as $100,000 per year per bullied nurse, and bullies usually have several targets. However, even if a bully targets only one nurse, the hostile practice environment impacts all staff and potentially affects the patients and families that nursing serves.

BEING A BULLY

In the literature on uncivil behavior in the academic or practice setting, the label "horizontal violence" is used to describe the behavior. However, Egues and Leinung (2013) inform us that horizontal violence is "simply bullying and abuse" (p. 186). In this chapter, I use the words *bully, bullies,* and *bullying* because they are terms that more graphically and accurately describe the horizontal violence phenomenon. *Bully,* as defined by *The Free Dictionary* (n.d.), is "a quarrelsome, overbearing person who badgers and intimidates weaker people." Bullies are chronically toxic individuals who seem to take joy in the act of bullying; however, they are generally quite careful to avoid bullying someone who will not take it.

How can a profession that is dedicated to caring, compassion, and the very human act of alleviating suffering in others allow the bully to inflict suffering on fellow nurses? Specifically, how can deans and healthcare administrators and managers not only overlook the human and financial costs of this mean-spirited and childish behavior, but also allow it to take hold in their organization's nursing culture? After this type of behavior has become embedded in a culture, it can take a herculean effort to remove it.

According to Gaardenfors (2006), humans only do what works for them to achieve their goals. In other words, bullying behavior works for the bully, and the behavior will continue until it no longer brings the bully benefit or reward. I suggest that a key benefit/reward for the chronic and habitual bully in academia and practice environments is that the bully very often gets to keep his or her job.

Bullying is well described in the literature, and it is not a new phenomenon. I believe that as individual nurses, and as a profession, we have long tolerated, ignored, witnessed, and encouraged bullying. Even worse, we may have participated in the act of bullying—either as a bully or as someone who has condoned the bullying behavior. Becher and Visovsky (2011), Freshwater (2000), Cooper et al. (2011), and Egues and Leinung (2013) indicate that bullying is the result of top-down-command-and-control academic and management practices, a lack of control over the clinical practice environment, low self-esteem, and a nursing history of being oppressed.

> *"The martyr sacrifices themselves entirely in vain. Or rather not in vain; for they make the selfish more selfish, the lazy more lazy, and the narrow narrower."*
>
> *–Florence Nightingale*

Although I completely understand how someone could be tempted to believe that bullying is an appropriate method for counteracting the preceding weaknesses, it does not excuse the behavior in any way. There is neither any valid excuse for becoming a bully, nor is there any excuse for allowing a bully to work in a healthcare or academic organization.

In 1977, as an early-career nurse, I quickly became very familiar with the act of "eating our young." I have often wondered where these cannibals learned their trade, and why we put up with them. Certainly, some bullies learned that behavior long before they arrived at nursing school. However, as academics, I believe that we must ask ourselves the following questions: "Have I contributed to, reinforced, or demonstrated bullying behavior toward other faculty in the presence of students?" and "Have I witnessed faculty-on-faculty, faculty-on-student, or student-on-student bullying?"

Cooper et al. (2011) note that faculty may not intentionally behave in ways that "demean or embarrass students" (p. 4). However, if you are the dean of faculty, it is ultimately your responsibility to inform bullies how their negative behavior contributes to a hostile learning environment. When bullying behavior is ignored, the leaders in the environment are communicating to students that this is acceptable behavior in nursing, and the people who exhibit the behavior act as role models. The bully should be provided with feedback and assistance to change; however, if the bullying behavior does not stop, my advice is to separate the culprit from the environment as quickly as possible.

Cooper et al., in their study on students' perceptions of bullying behaviors by nursing faculty, reported that school of nursing faculty were the most frequently reported source of bullying behaviors when "assigning course workload, changing clinical assignments, and giving a bad grade" (p. 12). Moreover, they identified that faculty used "belittling and humiliating behavior" as a bullying tactic. It is my strong belief that our students deserve better.

Herman (2011) notes that the best professors treat students as adults and offer them respect, as opposed to treating them as numbers on a class roster. Effective professors are accessible, apply class expectations equally to all students, and perhaps most important, have a passion for the topic and for teaching. They "go beyond the call of duty, know the material, and teach it well" (p. 2). Herman informs us that good professors maintain high expectations for all students and demonstrate a willingness to be flexible, meeting the students where they are and not where the faculty member hoped they would be.

Orlando (2013) expands on what Herman (2011) identifies as a good professor and describes him or her as someone who creates a sense of community and belonging in the classroom, is able to alter the teaching plan and methods when the lesson is not working, and models professionalism in all activities.

When a dean has knowledge that a bully is repeatedly assigned to work with students in any capacity but does nothing about it, the dean is the problem rather than the bully. From the student's perspective, the bully is there with the school's permission; therefore, students see very little chance of confronting the behaviors because they rightly fear recrimination.

When a school of nursing allows a known bully to graduate, the school is directly, and unambiguously, telling the practice environment that you tolerate this behavior. Although your school might not consider the behavior appropriate for a profession, because it has been tolerated, the school has contributed to the continuing problem of eating our young. Academics hold accountability for ensuring that student bullies do not become registered nurses.

Nursing faculty has the all-important role of welcoming the next generation of nurses into the profession, and the vast majority of nursing academics are wonderful role models. However, in carefully considering the number of faculty and students who may be affected by even a single negative role model, we see the impact is enormous.

The same is true for healthcare administrators who tolerate the chronic and habitual bully's presence. In 2007, the Joint Commission became so concerned about disruptive, uncivil, and bullying behaviors—because of their potential to create a hostile practice environment and the potential for patient harm—that it promulgated policies to combat uncivil behavior (Becher & Visovsky, 2012). If healthcare administrators and nurse leaders tolerate this behavior, the leaders are the problem because the bully is allowed to continue working. Because bullying has become such a problem in healthcare in general, and in nursing specifically, the ANA announced a position statement on zero tolerance for workplace bullying and violence on August 31, 2015. In a recent study, the ANA points out that up to 50% of the 3,765 nurses in the study had been bullied by a peer. Specifically, the ANA states: "The nursing profession will no longer tolerate violence of any kind from any source" (ANA, 2015a).

FUTURE FOCUS: CREATING OUR PREFERRED FUTURE

In 1995, Burton and Moran wrote the book *The Future Focused Organization: Complete Organizational Alignment for Breakthrough Results.* The authors provided organizations with a means to honor the past, to make the present as productive and progressive as possible, and to never lose sight that the future is where the future of an organization and its employees lies. The future rarely, if ever, knocks on your door and says, "Here is the key fob to the kingdom." You must discover your future.

○- - -▶

"We did not come to fear the future. We came here to shape it."
–Barack Obama

Just as individuals can suffer from paradigm paralysis, organizations can stagnate. They must learn to read the clues to the future, adapt accordingly, and not allow its paradigm to glue it to the present. The future-focused organization, as Burton and Moran (1995) remind us, is not "unwilling to sacrifice tomorrow on the altar of yesterday" (p. 1).

The idea of honoring our past, without allowing it to restrict our future, is of vital concern to any profession. Nursing must honor its past and use it as a foundation for progress while never allowing the past to totally define its future. Burton and Moran (1995) explain that the future-focused organization is constantly on a path of discovery; however, discovery is only one part of the process. The successful organization blends what it discovers with the organization's purpose to help guide its future. The future-focused organization listens, extracts, and adapts information from emerging thinkers (paradigm pioneers) from within and external to the profession to provide new building blocks that support the organization's purpose.

According to Burton and Moran (1995), the elements of a future-focused organization are its mission and purpose, its ability to have precision and clarity of purpose, and its ability to be specific about purpose, but not limiting in its application of its purpose. I believe these elements are applicable to the profession of nursing, which is constantly and specifically focused on identifying new opportunities and potentials for meeting the needs of all we serve and for meeting the needs of the profession's members.

> *"Change is the process by which the future invades our lives."*
> *—Alvin Toffler*

Applying Burton and Moran's (1995) model to the profession of nursing to keep it future-focused are (a) nursing's mission, primary concern, goals, and objectives, which are akin to the definition of nursing which clearly states why nurses exist; (b) nursing's ability to have precision and clarity about its purpose, which is akin to using evidence-based practice to improve our process and strategies for meeting the needs of all we serve, as well as the needs of the members of our profession; and (c) nursing must be specific about our mission but not limiting, which is akin to using our mission (definition of nursing) to expand nursing practice into areas not yet considered appropriate for nursing. To accomplish this, the profession must be willing to look to sources outside of nursing in an effort to improve how we meet the needs of all we serve. For instance, much of our work on safety has come from the manufacturing, airline, and nuclear industries.

Burton and Moran (1995) provide five additional strategies for success that nursing could adopt as a means of being future-focused:

- *Awareness, not unconsciousness*

  Awareness is the value that raises nursing's collective consciousness, cognitive powers, and self-fulfillment of its members.

- *Permissive, not dogmatic*

  Dogma is the clear path to destruction in any profession because it leads to the terminal disease of paradigm paralysis (Barker, 1992). This could prevent the profession from adequately responding to problems in real time, and also prevent the profession from effectively using the multiple and sometimes complex sources of feedback it receives.

- *Universal, not exclusionary*

  The need to understand the factors—internal and external— that contribute to overall success, knowing that the profession must continually scan our horizon(s) to identify factors that can facilitate growth. The balance between inclusion and exclusion is a delicate process. As mentioned earlier, not everyone should be a nurse.

- *Education, not training*

  Results and breakthrough improvements are not achieved by teaching techniques alone, or with just-in-time training.

Members of any profession must be *educated* to improve their thinking skills, and the occasional class is not robust enough to allow individuals within a profession to integrate learning into practice. If individuals do not integrate learning into their practice, then the collective wisdom and power of the nursing profession will be stymied.

- *Integration, not isolation*

  All professions must have a central nervous system that integrates, redirects, and sharpens the mission without creating silos that hinder progress at the individual and professional levels. The successful profession is not afraid of importing ideas, processes, and evidence from other professions to improve how it achieves its primary mission.

  Additionally, the efforts of nurse administrators and point-of-care nurses must become better integrated by using governance structures that bring them together in a respectful way to jointly solve the issues they face now and in the future.

PAY IT FORWARD

In order for any profession to be successful, its members must be willing to contribute to its future. One globally proven mechanism to accomplish this is the concept of *pay it forward (PIF)*. Needleman (2007) states, "Perhaps we see that no amount of getting can equal the genuine taste of giving" (p. 183).

PIF is a concept and practice that means when something good happens to you, you then do a good deed for someone else. Instead of paying it "backward" to the person who has helped you, the good deed is passed forward to someone else (InnovateUs, 2013). This method of kindness is infallible unless met with a greedy or an immature person (Inveterate, 2009).

The concept first appeared in U.S. popular literature and film in 2000, when Catherine Ryan Hyde's novel *Pay It Forward* was published and adapted into a film of the same name. Ryan Hyde describes PIF as the "obligation to do at least three good deeds for others in response to a good deed that you have received." A major lesson we can learn from PIF actions is that no matter how big problems might seem to us, each of us can make a difference in the lives of others, and it takes far less effort than one imagines.

An Internet search for PIF results in numerous associations and foundations that bring PIF to life—for example, the Pay It Forward Foundation (www.payitforwardfoundation.org). Pay It Forward Day was started in Australia by Blake Beattie in 2007 and has spread to more than 70 countries (Beattie, 2015). Thousands of websites explain the concept of PIF and provide suggestions for implementing it. A Google search for *nurses and pay it forward* generated tens of millions of hits. Numerous stories about nurses paying it forward are very inspiring and clearly demonstrate to the world that nurses are indeed worthy of being the most trusted profession in the United States (Riffkin, 2014).

The PIF actions in nursing are varied and dynamic and sometimes begin long before a nursing student arrives at school for the first day of class. PIF is a very rewarding experience and enables nurses to focus on what they can do in the present to improve their relationships with each other and with the patients, families, communities, and populations that nursing has the sacred and profound honor to serve.

In nursing, the first PIF opportunity is between students. Students have multiple opportunities to PIF with each other. For example, if you see a fellow student struggling with something that you have mastered, take the time to help the student to gain proficiency in that area. You might be helping a fellow student improve, thereby potentially preventing a clinical error. Moreover, your kindness can serve to demonstrate to your peer that we all have an obligation to assist others. Also, if students learn the importance of paying it forward in school, they are more likely to emerge into the practice arena ready and able to PIF with their professional colleagues.

PAYING IT FORWARD PROFESSIONALLY

In late 2015, two of my colleagues took time to respond to questions I had about the pay it forward concept and nursing. Erin Raney, BSN, CNML, is a nurse manager at NCH Healthcare in Naples, Florida; Marcia Sweasey, MSN, RN, is also a nurse manager at NCH Healthcare. Their thoughtful answers follow:

Crow: What does pay it forward mean to you as a person and a nurse?

Raney: As a person, paying it forward is an opportunity to do something kind for others. In nursing, paying it forward means improving areas of our profession, such as education and professional practice for current and future nurses. It is creating a better future for the nursing profession.

Sweasey: I was raised in a family of volunteers. It was expected to use the gifts you were given to help those less able or less fortunate. I carry the same philosophy in to my nursing practice. I was given a solid foundation as a young nurse, so it is my responsibility (and really my great joy) to help new nurses establish their practice, to facilitate their growth, and provide them with the resources to explore the many different avenues of our profession.

Crow: Where did the impulse to pay it forward come from—family, friends, other sources?

Raney: As a nurse we want to help people, including not only our patients but those in our profession or aspiring nurses. The impulse to pay it forward comes from a variety of sources. One of the sources is an internal desire to do good things for others. Paying it forward and giving back to others was also something that I was raised to do. Another source is from other nurse colleagues. Some of the best mentors I have had in my career have demonstrated and taught me the importance of giving back to others and improving our profession.

Sweasey: Definitely family influence, but solidly reinforced by close friends and church family. Most of the people I surround myself with share this philosophy of sharing gifts/talent/experience, so we support and inspire each other.

Crow: What benefits do you get from the pay-it-forward experience in Vietnam?

Raney: The Vietnam experience has given me a great deal of personal satisfaction. Personally, it is very rewarding to know that I have helped others. Professionally, I have learned best practices and new ideas from other nurse colleagues. It is also a wonderful thing to hear about and experience the excitement from the Vietnamese nurses when they learn best practices. They are inspired to do better for their patients and their profession, and they put their new knowledge into action.

Sweasey: Several things come to mind. The intense personal satisfaction in knowing that my skills and efforts had some small part in improving a child's life; sharing subject matter expertise and experiences to help improve nursing practice in an emerging nursing population; and the joy in realizing that while we have different skill levels as nurses, our common thread is that we care about others and want to do whatever needs to be done to ensure that those we care for achieve the best possible outcomes.

Crow: How did the VNP become the focus of pay it forward for NCH nursing?

Raney: When Marcia and I returned from our trip to Vietnam, our NCH colleagues were excited to hear about our trip and experience. Each year during Nurses' Week, a project or program is selected to be the recipient of donations collected during the week. This year VNP [Vietnam Nurse Project] was the program selected for our pay it forward initiative. Marcia and I created a story board about VNP and shared it at each Nurses' Week event.

Sweasey: I would have to say that it was your passion for this project that brought it to the forefront. The way you spoke about your experiences made me want to do the same. When we returned from the trip, we shared with any- and everyone who showed the slightest interest. We also had a great advocate in our ACNO, Laurie Zone Smith, who promoted our efforts to all. It was actually her idea to make VNP the focus of our Nurses' Week giving—encouraging the nurses at NCH to take a step out to help our sister nurses in Vietnam.

As a realistic optimist, my glass is simultaneously half-empty and half-full. There are times in my career when I have been an optimist about nursing, but not about nurses, and vice versa. Like most nurses that I have practiced with, the art and science of our practice are important to me. When workload does not exceed resources, nurses have the opportunity to truly think about how to combine the art and science of our practice. Yet, at other times, I have experienced the profession at its worst, and I felt crushed by the overwhelming needs that surrounded me. The all-too-familiar burden of feeling like there is too much to accomplish with too little time or resources can indefinitely delay, or even block, any hope of advocating for a brighter future for the nurse or the profession of nursing.

COLLECTIVE INTELLIGENCE

Because we are knowledge professionals, it is critical that we in the nursing profession establish governance structures and processes that allow opportunities for nurses to step away from the day-to-day accountabilities of direct patient care. We need to be given time to think about nursing so that we can consider ways that we can improve nursing care and nourish our profession.

Nurses' participation in shared governance structures will enable us as point-of-care nurses to assess and identify needs, and to propose, implement, and evaluate the impact of evidence-based solutions as they pertain to nursing care and practice. It is important to understand that "nursing care" and "the care of nursing" are not the same.

Dock and Stewart (1931) state, "If a group is to put forth its utmost effort it must have a normal outlet for its intelligence and initiative as well as *its spirit of service*" (p. 345). The normal outlet of nursing has been traditionally thought of as bedside care. However, it has been my experience that all nurses—whether working in the United States or in other developed or developing countries—have very little time to consider the future of nursing or how to improve it locally while being simultaneously focused on the immediate needs of those for whom they are providing care.

It is imperative that we shift our thinking about what is a normal outlet for nursing and focus our efforts on our collective intelligence. Nurses must be allocated time to think about nursing care and the care of nursing. The work of thinking about practice development *is* nursing practice.

AN ADVOCATE FOR NURSING

Advocacy is defined as "the act of pleading or arguing in favor of something such as a cause, idea, or policy" (The Free Dictionary, n.d.). The central idea is to work on behalf of others or one's self, to raise awareness about a concern, and to promote evidence-based solutions to the issue. A proposal without evidence or data to support it is not worth proposing.

One must be prepared when assuming the role of advocate. As Rogers (2003) argues, the advocate, or any change agent, must make the case that the policy being advocated is perceived as superior to the one it is replacing. Advocates, paradigm pioneers, and change agents must learn the art and science of marketing ideas, and they also must have the ability to communicate their ideas in a language the audience will understand, preferably in 60 seconds or less.

60-SECOND SPEECHES

Tomajan (2012) provides a model for how to craft a short, concise, and informative 60-second presentation:

- Share your name, where you practice and live, and the name of the department or agency you are representing.
- Describe the issue you are addressing.
- Put a human face on your request, paint a word picture, and/or tell a story.
- Describe what you would like for the person/group to do.
- Distribute a fact sheet describing your request and including your contact information.

Source: Tomajan, K. (2012). Advocating for nurses and nursing. *The Online Journal of Issues in Nursing, 17*(1), 1–12.

Most of the advocacy activities in nursing have been focused on methods of safe and effective nursing care. Advocacy for the profession of nursing has been mostly left up to nursing associations (Benton, 2012). Benton informs us that from his perspective as CEO of the International Council of Nurses (ICN), most of the advances in nursing have been the product of nursing associations, of which the ICN is one example.

Benton (2012) also notes that "the single most important factor in influencing healthcare sector policy is solidarity within the profession… Unity within the profession is essential to ensure that nursing's voice is heard" (p. 4). However, little progress could be accomplished if the leaders of these nursing associations did not have a clear and concise vision when advocating for nursing.

Tomajan (2012) notes that advocacy often requires that the work be done via formal decision-making bodies to achieve a desired outcome. However, many point-of-care nurses view the formal decision-making bodies—which are often in the upper levels of the organization—as a black hole where great ideas die.

POINT OF CARE NURSE ADVOCATE

Nurses at the point of care (POC) play an important advocacy role within their organizations and in the nursing profession. According to Tomajan (2012), to ensure some modicum of success, advocates and change agents must "possess in good measure the skills of problem-solving, communication, influence, and collaboration" (p. 3). As POC nurses develop and apply their advocacy skills, they are better able to promote a positive practice environment and to improve the profession.

Organizations must design and implement shared power structures that provide opportunities for nurses to work collaboratively with management to solve problems. The power structure must consist of decentralized bodies, sometimes referred to as "councils," that are empowered to make evidence-based decisions within the council's scope of accountability that has been outlined in the organization's bylaws. Councils must be chaired, and co-chaired, by POC nurses. All council members are responsible for representing the needs of their colleagues, their patients, and the profession as a whole (Tomajan, 2012). It is an expectation that POC nurses will role model professional behavior, precept new graduate nurses, and help to inform the public about what nurses do to promote and protect public health (Tomajan, 2012).

MANAGER/ADMINISTRATOR NURSE ADVOCATE

One of the most important roles for the nurse manager/administrator is to protect, or improve, the number of resources available for the POC nurses (Tomajan, 2012). Furthermore, it is vital for leaders to involve nurses in resource allocation and also in resource management. It is important for POC nurses to know the cost of the care they are providing and to continuously strive to improve quality and patient outcomes while conserving as many resources as possible. Without cost-of-care information, the POC nurses cannot collaborate in a productive way to manage the resources in the best interest of their patients and the organization.

Managers and administrators must advocate for the design, implementation, and maintenance of power-sharing structures, such as shared governance. A central tenet of shared governance is to involve those affected by a proposed change in the design, implementation, and evaluation of potential solutions. The sharing of power among managers/administrators and POC nurses has the potential to co-evolve nursing. Kelly (1994) informs us that "evolution is adapting to meet one's needs, and co-evolution is adapting to meet each other's needs" (p. 74). Co-evolution cannot occur with top-down-command-and-control, or secrecy. In fact, co-evolution is the work of nursing's future.

NURSE EDUCATORS AS ADVOCATES

Nursing faculty play one of the most vital roles in nourishing the next generation of nurse colleagues and in creating a student's identity as a nurse. The initial conditions under which a new nursing student receives his or her education will greatly affect the student's identity as a nurse. Tomajan (2012) posits that, "Faculty in academic settings and nurse educators in professional development roles serve as the culture carriers of the profession" (p. 9). Educators can create a sense of belonging for students, which becomes fundamental to their success. Walker et al. (2014) note that belongingness helps to establish a collegial relationship between student and faculty, and it is a "fundamental precursor to active learning and development" (p. 103). An important role of nurse educators in academia and practice is to constantly scan the environment within, and outside of, healthcare to identify products and processes that will enhance the ability of nurses to meet the needs of those they serve.

PERSONAL APPLICATION

The following questions are designed to help you reflect on the knowledge and wisdom you have gained over your career and to facilitate the successful transfer of this knowledge and wisdom to those nurse leaders who, like you, have devoted their life's work to their patients and to the nursing profession.

1. Identify the sources of your professional identity.
   - Who has been the most influential person in the formation of your professional identity?
   - How did nursing school influence your professional identity?
   - Did your undergraduate, master's, or doctoral program have the greatest impact on your professional identity? Explain.

2. Paradigm paralysis can block the development of nursing as a profession.
   - In what ways has paradigm paralysis hindered the development of nursing practice where you currently practice?
   - How would you help your boss understand that her/his paradigm of nursing is outdated and harming nursing where you practice?

3. The selection process for hiring can help or hinder nursing.
   - What are the major criteria your organization uses to screen and hire healthcare professionals?
   - How does your organization deal with bullies?
   - When you decide to separate a bully from your organization, where do you get the greatest support, and what is the source of the least amount of support?

4. In nursing, "eating our young" is a well-documented phenomenon.

    • How would you describe the most blatant example of a nurse eating our young that you have personally witnessed?

    • From your perspective, what is the impact of eating our young on your organization and the nursing profession?

5. Future-focused organizations are not willing to sacrifice tomorrow on the altar of yesterday.

    • How do you help your colleagues see that change is the work of nursing?

    • When your colleagues are stuck in the past, how do you assist them in updating their paradigm of nursing?

6. To pay it forward, one must be willing to offer a gift while expecting nothing in return.

    • In what ways have you role-modeled pay it forward with students, colleagues, and your organization?

    • How have you influenced mentees to pay it forward?

7. Power-sharing structures and processes such as shared governance can increase staff engagement.

    • Has your organization designed and implemented a power-sharing model? If yes, how effective is that model in solving major problems faced by your organization?

    • What are the major impediments to the implementation of a power-sharing model in your organization?

    • What are the major benefits of power sharing to the development of the nursing profession?

LOOKING FORWARD

All nurses throughout the world have the professional obligation to improve nursing where they practice. We must stand together in an effort to have our collective voices heard and to help shape healthcare around the world. Standing together means that we must welcome the next generation of nurses into our profession in a way that makes them feel that they belong in nursing.

While my generation of nurses has not solved all of nursing's woes, we have made great strides in many areas. It is now up to the next generation of nurses to take up the mantle of progress and to improve the nursing profession in ways that will amaze future nurses, the healthcare environments in which they practice, and the public they serve. Today's nurses have tools that were not readily available to past generations, and those tools will enable them to, as Dock and Stewart (1931) tell us, not fall back or hinder the development of our profession but always move it forward.

AFTERWORD

Successful leaders, like all of us, have only one life in which to share their wisdom, experience, and knowledge. Books, particularly textbooks, have a tendency to fade away, although they are often quoted in scholarly papers. During that one lifetime authentic leaders have the accountability—not just the responsibility—to assure continuity of knowledge for those who come after. Kathy Malloch and Tim Porter-O'Grady have captured the essence of critical leadership functions: the transference of knowledge and succession management.

Malloch and Porter-O'Grady's outstanding work in integrating innovation, evidence-based practice (EBP), and succession planning is nothing less than brilliant. Their commitment to sharing, mentoring, and coaching and assuring that their work and the work of others lives on is outstanding. Individual authors share different perspectives while recognizing that nurses share their knowledge about patients skillfully and have the innate ability to share their wisdom as well. The well-thought-out concern about many current leaders who are retiring and the need for them to share as well cannot be overstated.

Meaningful communication is one of the critical foundations of professionalism. In these hectic times of transition, it is more important than ever that our wisdom leaders share.

The continuing remarkable work that is done by Malloch and Porter-O'Grady will live on. This amazing book assures that the work they have contributed to nursing and healthcare will not be overlooked. This exceptional book has so much to offer that an afterword cannot do it justice.

–Roxane Spitzer, PHD, RN, MBA, MA, FAAN
Editor in Chief, *Nurse Leader*
Vice President, Strategy, OnSomble

REFERENCES AND RECOMMENDED READING

CHAPTER 1

REFERENCES

Brockbank, A., & McGill, I. (2012). *Facilitating reflective learning: Coaching, mentoring and supervision*. Retrieved from http://www.columbia.edu/cgi-bin/cul/resolve?clio10039489

Brown, A. (2014). Organizational paradigms and sustainability in excellence: From mechanistic approaches to learning and innovation. *International Journal of Quality and Service Sciences, 6*(2), 181–190.

Burton-Jones, A., & Spender, J. C. (2011). *The Oxford handbook of human capital*. Oxford handbooks in business and management. Oxford, UK: Oxford University Press: 1 online resource (xviii, 6888 pages).

Franklin, B. (n.d.). Retrieved from http://www.goodreads.com/author/quotes/289513. Benjamin_Franklin

Frost, R. (n.d.). Retrieved from http://www.goodreads.com/author/show/7715.Robert_Frost

Malloch, K., & Porter-O'Grady, T. (2010). *The quantum leader: Applications for the new world of work*. Boston, MA: Jones & Bartlett.

McKay, D. O. (n.d.). Retrieved from http://www.goodreads.com/author/show/601416. David_O_McKay

Patton, R., Zalon, M., & Ludwick, R. (Eds.). (2015). *Nurses making policy: From bedside to boardroom*. New York, NY: Springer.

Piper, L. E. (2012). Generation Y in healthcare: Leading millennials in an era of reform. *Frontiers of Health Services Management, 29*(1), 16–28.

Plutarch. (n.d.). Retrieved from http://www.goodreads.com/author/show/31015. Plutarch

Raes, E., Decuyper, S., & Lismont, B. (2013). Facilitating team learning through transformational leadership. *Instructional Science, 41*(2), 287–305.

Swanwick, T., & McKimm, J. (2011). *ABC of clinical leadership.* Chichester, West Sussex, UK: BMJ Books.

CHAPTER 2

REFERENCES

Adams, L. (2011). Learning a new skill is easier said than done. Gordon Training International. Retrieved from http://www.gordontraining.com/free-workplace-articles/learning-a-new-skill-is-easier-said-than-done

American Organization of Nurse Executives. (2013). AONE salary and compensation study for nurse leaders. Washington, DC: Author.

Boychuk-Duchscher, J. E., & Cowin, L. (2004). Multi-generational nurses in the workplace. *Journal of Nursing Administration, 34*(11), 493–501.

Bridges, W. (2009). *Managing transitions: Making the most of change.* Philadelphia, PA: Da Capo Press.

Kutin, J. (2012). Distinct generations make nursing leadership challenging. Retrieved from http://www.nursetogether.com/distinct-generations-make-nursing-leadership-challenging

Larkin, H. (2015). The traits of today's ideal health care CEO. *H&HN.* Retrieved from http://www.hhnmag.com/Magazine/2015/June/cover-new-health-care-CEO

MacMillan, D. (2008). Issue: Retiring employees, lost knowledge. Retrieved from http://www.bloomberg.com/bw/stories/2008-08-20/issue-retiring-employees-lost-knowledgebusinessweek-business-news-stock-market-and-financial-advice

McGraw, Mark. (2013). A mass exodus of millennials? Retrieved from http://www.hreonline.com/HRE/view/story.jhtml?id=534355895

McMenamin, P. (2014). 2022: Where have all those nurses gone? Retrieved from http://www.ananursespace.org/blogs/peter-mcmenamin/2014/03/14/rn-retirements-tsunami-warning?ssopc=1

Sherman, R. (2013). What competencies do nurse leaders need today? Retrieved from http://www.emergingrnleader.com/competenciesnurseleadersneed

Society for Human Resource Management. (2014). Executive summary: Preparing for an aging workforce. Retrieved from https://www.shrm.org/Research/SurveyFindings/Documents/14-0765%20Executive%20Briefing%20Aging%20Workforce%20v4.pdf

Tzyh-Lih, H., Lin, L., Wu, J., & Tsai, H. (2006). A framework for designing nursing knowledge systems. *Interdisciplinary Journal of Information, Knowledge, and Management, 1*(1), 13–22.

CHAPTER 3

REFERENCES

Balanced Scorecard Institute. (n.d.). Balanced scorecard basics. Retrieved from https://balancedscorecard.org/Resources/About-the-Balanced-Scorecard

Centers for Medicare & Medicaid Services. (2015). Background. Retrieved from www.hcahpsonline.org

Collins, J. (2001). *Good to great*. New York, NY: HarperCollins.

EntrepreneurWiki.com. (n.d.). Caterina Fake. Retrieved from http://entrepreneurwiki.com/EW/Caterina_Fake

FindLaw. (2013). How to write a business contract. Retrieved from http://smallbusiness.findlaw.com/business-contracts-forms/how-to-write-a-business-contract.html

Frankel, A. (2009). Nurses' learning styles: Promoting better integration of theory into practice. *Nursing Times, 105*(2), 24–27.

Giang, V. (2013). 7 email etiquette rules every professional should know. *Business Insider*. Retrieved from http://www.businessinsider.com/email-etiquette-rules-barbara-pachter-2013-10#ixzz3aWhpWezX

Kaplan, R. S., & Norton, D. P. (1996). Using the balanced scorecard as a strategic management system. *Harvard Business Review, 74*(1), 75–85.

National Patient Safety Foundation. (2015). Ask me 3. Retrieved from http://www.npsf.org/?page=askme3

Shirley, R. (2010). How do you learn? Retrieved from http://www.worldwidelearn.com/education-articles/how-do-you-learn.htm

CHAPTER 4

REFERENCES

Blanchard, K. (2015). How we help. Retrieved from http://www.kenblanchard.com/government/How-We-Help

Coleman, J. (2012, August 15). For those who want to lead, read. *Harvard Business Review*. Retrieved from https://hbr.org/2012/08/for-those-who-want-to-lead-rea

Collins, J. (2001). *Good to great. Why some companies make the leap ... and others don't*. New York, NY: HarperCollins.

Covey, S. (1989). *The 7 habits of highly effective people: Powerful lessons in personal change*. New York, NY: Fireside.

Drucker, P. F. (1996). *The leader of the future*. Hoboken, NJ: Wiley.

Dunn, P. (2005, October 7). 4 ways to present your information – Dale Carnegie's prescient advice. Retrieved from http://www.qualitywriter.com/2005/4-ways-to-present-your-information-dale-carnegies-prescient-advice

Johnson, S. (2002). *Who moved my cheese? An a-mazing way to deal with change in your work and in your life*. New York, NY: G. P. Putnam's Sons.

Tjan, A. K. (2010, August 9). The power of ignorance. *Harvard Business Review*. Retrieved from https://hbr.org/2010/08/the-power-of-ignorance.html

Welch, J. (2015, May 20). A collection of quotes from Jack Welch. Retrieved from http://www.slideshare.net/optimaltransformation/collection-of-quotes-from-jack-welch

CHAPTER 5

REFERENCES

Ackoff, R. L. (1989). From data to wisdom. *Journal of Applied Systems Analysis, 16*, 3–9.

Aristotle. (n.d.). Retrieved from https://www.goodreads.com/author/quotes/2192.Aristotle

Armstrong, T. (n.d.). Howard Gardner's theory of multiple intelligences. Retrieved from http://www.niu.edu/facdev/resources/guide/learning/howard_gardner_theory_multiple_intelligences.pdf

Baumlin, J. S. (1987). Persuasion, rogerian rhetoric, and imaginative play. *Rhetoric Society Quarterly, 17*(1), 33–43.

Brent, D. (1996). Rogerian rhetoric: An alternative to traditional rhetoric. In Barbara Emmel, Paula Resch, & Deborah Tenny (Eds.), *Argument revisited, argument redefined: Negotiating meaning in the composition classroom* (pp. 73–96). Thousand Oaks, CA: SAGE Publications.

Cerbin, W. (2011). Understanding learning styles: A conversation with Dr. Bill Cerbin. Interview with Nancy Chick. Virtual Teaching and Learning Center of the University of Wisconsin Colleges.

Chick, N. (2015). Learning styles. Retrieved from http://cft.vanderbilt.edu/guides-sub-pages/learning-styles-preferences

Frank, C. J., & Magnone, P. (2011). *Drinking from the fire hose: Making smarter decisions without drowning in information.* New York, NY: Penguin.

Haggard, S. (2010). Stand up for yourself or bite your tongue - How to pick your battles at work. Ezine @rticles. Retrieved from http://ezinearticles.com/? Stand-Up-For-Yourself-Or-Bite-Your-Tongue---How-to-Pick-Your-Battles-at-Work&id=4344489

Herodotus. (n.d.). Retrieved from https://www.goodreads.com/author/quotes/901.Herodotus

Information. (n.d.). In *Business Dictionary*. Retrieved from http://www.businessdictionary.com/definition/information.html

James, J. (2012). How much data is created every minute? Retrieved from https://www.domo.com/blog/2012/06/how-much-data-is-created-every-minute

Lang, A. (n.d.). Retrieved from https://www.goodreads.com/author/quotes/18393.Andrew_Lang

National Research Council. (1999). A question of balance: Private rights and the public interest in scientific and technical databases. Washington, DC: National Academies Press. Retrieved from http://www.nap.edu/openbook.php?record_id=9692

O'Brien, T., Bernold, L. E., & Akroyd, D. (1998). Myers-Briggs type indicator and academic achievement in engineering education. *International Journal of Engineering Education, 14*(5), 311–315.

Plato. (n.d.). Retrieved from https://www.goodreads.com/author/quotes/879.Plato

Reed, M. G. (2010, February 25). Data deluge. *The Economist*, pp. 10–12.

Scuderi, R. (n.d.). What are the differences between knowledge, wisdom, and insight? Retrieved from http://www.lifehack.org/articles/communication/what-are-the-differences-between-knowledge-wisdom-and-insight.html

Siegler, M. G. (2010). Eric Schmidt: Every 2 days we create as much information as we did up to 2003. Retrieved from http://techcrunch.com/2010/08/04/schmidt-data

Strauss, W., & Howe, N. (1997). *The fourth turning: An American prophecy - what the cycles of history tell us about America's next rendezvous with destiny.* New York, NY: Broadway Books.

Tanner, K., & Allen, D. (Winter 2004). Approaches to biology teaching and learning: Learning styles and the problem of instructional selection-engaging all students in science courses. *Cell Biology Education, 3*(4), 197–201.

von Goethe, J. W. (n.d.). Retrieved from http://www.brainyquote.com/quotes/quotes/j/johannwolf382514.html

Young, R. E., Becker, A. L., & Pike, K. L. (1970). *Rhetoric: Discovery and change.* New York, NY: Harcourt.

CHAPTER 6

REFERENCES

Celebrate. (n.d.). In *Merriam-Webster's online dictionary.* Retrieved from http://www.merriam-webster.com/thesaurus/celebrate

Collaboration. (n.d.). In *Wikipedia.* Retrieved September 2, 2015, from http://en.wikipedia.org/wiki/Collaboration

Inskeep, S., & Groopman, J. (2007, March 16). Groopman: The doctor's in, but is he listening? In S. Inskeep (Producer), *Morning Edition.* Philadelphia, PA: National Public Radio. Retrieved from http://www.npr.org/2007/03/16/8946558/groopman-the-doctors-in-but-is-he-listening

Kimsey-House, H., Kimsey-House, K., Sandahl, P., & Whitworth, L. (2011). *Co-active coaching: Changing business, transforming lives* (3rd ed.). Boston, MA: Nicholas Brealey Publishing.

Kunich, J. C., & Lester, R. I. (1999). Leadership and the art of mentoring: Tool kit for the time machine. *The Journal of Leadership & Organizational Studies, 6*(1–2), 17–35.

Recognition. (n.d.). In *Merriam-Webster's online dictionary.* Retrieved from http://www.merriam-webster.com/dictionary/recognition

Relationship. (n.d.). In *The Free Dictionary.* Retrieved from http://www.thefreedictionary.com/relationship

Rhoades, D. R., McFarland, K. F., Finch, W. H., & Johnson, A. O. (2001). Speaking and interruptions during primary care office visits. *Family Medicine, 33*(7), 528–532.

Senge, P., Roberts, C., Ross, R. B., Smith, B. J., & Kleiner, A. (1994). *The fifth discipline fieldbook: Strategies and tools for building a learning organization.* New York, NY: Doubleday.

Sole, D., & Wilson, D. G. (2002). Storytelling in organizations: The power and traps of using stories to share knowledge in organization. Harvard Graduate School of Education. Retrieved from http://www.providersedge.com/docs/km_articles/storytelling_in_organizations.pdf

Stoltzfus, T. (2002). *Coaching questions: A coach's guide to powerful asking skills.* Virginia Beach, VA: Coach 22.

Trautman, S. (2014, August 22). The myth of the knowledge-hoarding expert unwilling to mentor peers. [Blog post]. Retrieved from http://www.hr.com/en/app/blog/2014/08/the-myth-of-the-knowledge-hoarding-expert-unwillin_hz69a2hx.html

Whitworth, L., Kimsey-House, K., Kimsey-House, H., & Sandahl, P. (2007). *Co-active coaching: New skills for coaching people toward success in work and life.* Mountain View, CA: Davies-Black Publishing.

RECOMMENDED READING

American College of Healthcare Executives. (2001–2003). Mentorship documents. Retrieved from www.ache.org

Jackson Leadership Systems. (2001). The power of mentoring. *Leadership Review.*

Reamy, T. (2002, June). Imparting knowledge through storytelling, part 1. *KMWorld, 11*(6). Retrieved from http://www.kmworld.com/Articles/Editorial/Features/Imparting-knowledge-through-storytelling-Part-1-of-a-two-part-article-9358.aspx

Reamy, T. (2002, July). Imparting knowledge through storytelling, part 2. *KMWorld, 11*(7). Retrieved from http://www.kmworld.com/Articles/Editorial/Features/Imparting-knowledge-through-storytelling-Part-2-9374.aspx

Rothwell, W. J. (2004). Capturing the lessons of experience: Knowledge transfer: 12 strategies for succession management. *IPMA-HR News*, February 2004, 10–11.

Thielfoldt, D. (2014). Passing the torch: Transferring knowledge from baby boomer employees to the next generation(s). *Insulation Outlook*. Retrieved from http://www.insulation.org/io/article.cfm?id=IO140202

CHAPTER 7

REFERENCES

The American Council on Education. (2015). First report: Reinvesting in the third age: Older adults and higher education. Retrieved from http://fliphtml5.com/liuu/nlfz/basic

Centers for Disease Control and Prevention. (2013). The state of aging and health in America. Atlanta, GA: U.S. Department of Health and Human Services.

Corporation for National and Community Service. (2013). Retrieved from http://www.volunteeringinamerica.gov/rankings/States/Baby-Boomer`-Volunteer-Rates/2011

Crawford, D. L. (2004). The role of aging in adult learning. Johns Hopkins School of Education. Retrieved from http://education.jhu.edu/PD/newhorizons/lifelonglearning/higher-education/implications

Gandhi, M. (n.d.). Mahatma Gandhi quotes. Retrieved from https://www.goodreads. com/quotes/2253-live-as-if-you-were-to-die-tomorrow-learn-as

Heller, N. (2011, July 29). Book clubs: Why do we love them so much? Is it the zucchini bread? Retrieved from http://www.slate.com/articles/news_and_politics/ assessment/2011/07/book_clubs.html

MacArthur Foundation. (2008). The MacArthur Research Network on an Aging Society. Retrieved from www.macfound.org/media/article_pdfs/AGING-INFOSHEET.PDF

Marx, G. (n.d.). Groucho Marx quotes. Retrieved from http://thinkexist.com/quotes/ groucho_marx

Quotes.net. (n.d.). "By learning you will teach…" Retrieved from http://www.quotes. net/quote/16678

Spiers, P. (2012). *Master class: Living longer, stronger, and happier.* New York, NY: Hachette/Center Street.

Tolkien, J. R. R. (n.d.). J. R. R. Tolkien quotes. Retrieved from https://www.goodreads. com/author/show/656983.J_R_R_Tolkien

CHAPTER 8

REFERENCES

Advocacy. (n.d.). In *The Free Dictionary.* Retrieved from http://www.thefreedictionary. com/advocacy

American Nurses Association. (2015a). Position statement on incivility, bullying, and workplace violence. Retrieved from http://www.nursingworld.org/Bullying-Workplace-Violence

American Nurses Association. (2015b). What is nursing? Retrieved from Nursingworld.org/EspeciallyForYou/What-is-Nursing

Barker, J. A. (1992). *Paradigms: The business of discovering the future.* New York, NY: Harper Business.

Beattie, B. (2015). About the day. Retrieved from http://payitforwardday.com/about/ about-the-day

Becher, J., & Visovsky, C. (2012). Horizontal violence in nursing. *MEDSURG Nursing, 21*(4), 210–232.

Benton, D. (2012). Advocating globally to shape policy and strengthen nursing's influence. *The Online Journal of Issues in Nursing, 1*(1), 1–10.

Bully. (n.d.). In *The Free Dictionary.* Retrieved from http://www.thefreedictionary.com/ bully

Burton, T. T., & Moran, J. W. (1995). *The future focused organization: Complete organizational alignment for breakthrough results.* Englewood Cliffs, NJ: Prentice-Hall.

Cooper, R. M., Walker, J., Askew, R., Robinson, J. C., & McNair, M. (2011). Students' perceptions of bullying behaviors by nursing faculty. *Issues in Educational Research, 21*(2), 1–16.

Dock, L. L., & Stewart, I. M. (1931). *A short history of nursing: From the earliest time to the present day.* New York, NY: Putnam's & Sons.

Egues, A. L., & Leinung, E. Z. (2013). The bully within and without: Strategies to address horizontal violence in nursing. *Nursing Forum, 48*(3), 185–190.

Freshwater, D. (2000). Crosscurrents: Against cultural narration in nursing. *Journal of Advanced Nursing, 32*(2), 1–8.

Fuller, R. B. (n.d.). Retrieved from https://www.goodreads.com/author/quotes/11515303.R_Buckminster_Fuller

Gärdenfors, P. (2007). *How homo became sapiens.* New York, NY: Oxford Press.

Hammarskjold, D. (n.d.). Retrieved from http://www.brainyquote.com/quotes/quotes/d/daghammars162384.html

Herman, R. L. (2011). What makes a good professor? *The Journal of Effective Teaching, 11*(1), 1–5.

InnovateUs. (2013). What does the idiom "pay it forward" mean? Retrieved from www.innovateus.net/innopedia/what-does-idiom-pay-it-forward-mean

Kelly, K. (1994). *Out of control: The new biology of machines, social systems, and the economic world.* New York, NY: Addison-Wesley.

Needleman, J. (2007). *Why can't we be good?* New York, NY: Penguin.

Nightingale, F. (n.d.). Retrieved from http://www.brainyquote.com/quotes/quotes/f/florenceni159064.html

Nightingale, F. (1969). *Notes on nursing: What it is and what it is not.* New York, NY: Dover Publications.

Obama, B. (n.d.). Retrieved from http://www.notable-quotes.com/o/obama_barack_x.html

Orlando, M. (2013). Nine characteristics of a great teacher. Retrieved from http://www.facultyfocus.com/articles/philosophy-of-teaching/nine-characteristics-of-a-great-teacher

Pay it forward. (2009). In *Urban Dictionary.* Retrieved from www.urbandictionary.com/payitforward

Riffkin, R. (2014). Americans rate nurses highest on honesty, ethical standards. Gallup.com. Retrieved from http://www.gallup.com/poll/180260/americans-rate-nurses-highest-honesty-ethical-standards.aspx

Rogers, E. M. (2003). *Diffusion of innovation* (5th ed.). New York, NY: Free Press.

Toffler, A. (n.d.). Retrieved from http://www.managementgurus.org/Alvin+Toffler

Tomajan, K. (2012). Advocating for nurses and nursing. *The Online Journal of Issues in Nursing, 1*(1), 1–12.

Walker, S., Dwyer, T., Broadbent, M., Moxham, L., Sander, T., & Edwards, K. (2014). Constructing a nursing identity within the clinical environment: The student nurse perspective. *Contemporary Nurse, 49*(1), 103–112.

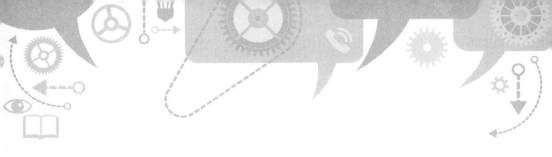

INDEX

L

M

The Mastering Series:
Handbooks for Success

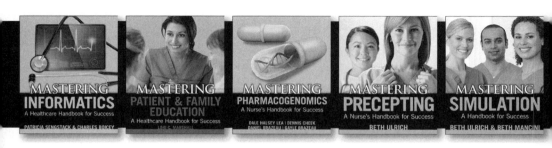

Mastering Informatics	Mastering Patient & Family Education	Mastering Pharmaco-genomics	Mastering Precepting	Mastering Simulation
Patricia Sengstack and Charles Boicey	Lori C. Marshall	Dale Halsey Lea, Dennis Cheek, Daniel Brazeau, and Gayle Brazeau	Beth Ulrich	Beth Ulrich and Beth Mancini

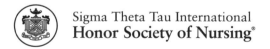

Sigma Theta Tau International
Honor Society of Nursing®

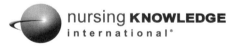

nursing **KNOWLEDGE**
international®

Resources for Clinical Leaders

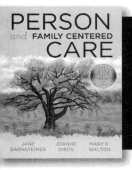

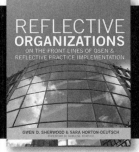

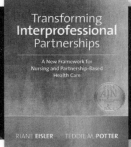

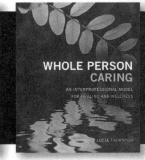

Person and Family
Centered Care

Jane Barnsteiner, Joanne
Disch, and Mary K. Walton

Reflective
Organizations

Gwen D. Sherwood and
Sara Horton-Deutsch

Transforming
Interprofessional
Partnerships

Riane Eisler and
Teddie M. Potter

Whole Person
Caring

Lucia Thornton

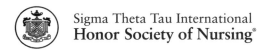

Sigma Theta Tau International
Honor Society of Nursing®

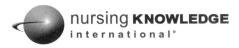

nursing **KNOWLEDGE**
i n t e r n a t i o n a l®

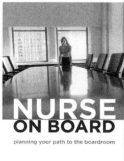

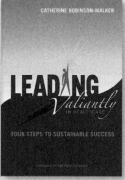
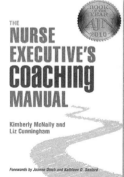
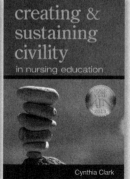

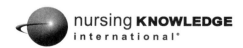